The Cancer Chronicles

Trey R. Barker

The Cancer Chronicles

Copyright © 2010 by Trey R. Barker

Cover design copyright © 2010
Brokaw Imagination
www.brokawimagination.com

First printing: April, 2010
ISBN: 978-0-557-35322-4

This is for all the local cops – especially the Bureau County Sheriff's Office and the Princeton Police Department – who helped me get through the nightmare that was a year sucking down chemo. I would never have made it through without you guys, and I'll never be able to say thanks enough.

But it's also for my wife LuAnn, who lived it with me, and Ben Atkinson, who laughed it with me. Together, you two managed to keep me alive and sane.

Part 1
November 27, 2005 – 1:51 pm

An odd thing, to be told you have cancer.

It was a simple thing. I had a bit of swelling on the right side of my neck. Like an infected lymph node, or swollen glands from a cold or flu. Went to the doc, got some antibiotics, swelling went away. A few weeks later, it came back and I got some heavier duty antibiotics. Swelling went away.

Then it came back.

In early September, sitting in a bar in Chicago with novelist Sean Doolittle, I can remember him eyeing the swelling and making a subdued comment. No problem, I told him. Gonna get it checked out when I get home.

A bit after that, I went back to my doc. I've never seen a man's eyes as big as his when he saw the swelling. It was blueberry-sized, maybe a bit larger. Pressing so hard against the nerves in my neck I had to take a few days off from the Sheriff's Office. He gave me some steroids and hooked me up with a surgeon. Said surgeon didn't seem overly concerned. He gave me lots and lots of statistics about how a swelling in that area almost always meant nothing. In fact, he rescheduled my surgery for two weeks after the original date because he was going to be out of town.

Not worried at all.

The surgery went fine, he said he got the entire lymph node and everything looked clean. A few days later, my regular doctor called and asked me to come in. He casually mentioned that I should go see an oncologist.

"So there was a problem?" I asked, slightly confused and now suddenly sweaty and hot, my gut tight as a snare drum.

"The biopsy came back as malignant melanoma."

And with that, I was ushered in to an entirely new world. One of stage 3 cancer and Interferon treatments and early diagnosis and 80 percent recurrence rates and endless weeks of weakness from chemo and — worse yet — pity from people around me.

The pity is not the worst. The worst, obviously, is the possibility of dying way sooner than I'd like (but isn't that a possibility pretty much every day? In a world of random shootings, heart attacks, drunk drivers, strokes, etc.) But seeing the eyes of people who suddenly don't know what to say is more than a little disconcerting.

They roll out all the platitudes. "Jeez, dude, I hope everything comes out okay."

Uh, yeah, me, too!

"You'll be fine, don't worry about it."

Uh, yeah, no problem, won't worry at all. It only kills how many people a year? But, yeah, I won't sweat it.

Honestly, I'd just as soon they shut the fuck up. If you're not sure what to say, don't say anything.

But in the midst of the maddening, superficial words, there were two friends who made me laugh my ass off. I called Sean, the novelist I mentioned earlier, to let him know what was going on. He had had my new novel for a little while, reading and critiquing it. When I got him on the phone, I basically got this from him: "Dude, you have cancer? Wow, that's too bad because your novel sucks, too."

(A disclaimer: the conversation didn't go exactly like that, but that's the funniest way to tell the story...writer's license and all that.)

The other was a guy I've gotten to know decently well only in the last few months. Ben Atkinson, a sergeant with the Princeton Police Department. He and I talked quite a bit about what was going on with me. He took me to lunch one day and told me straight out he was worried about me. Worried about the depression I was going through in the two or three days after the diagnosis.

Standing in the parking lot after lunch, he said, "I'm just worried," and mimicked putting a gun in his mouth.

Uh…what?

Yeah, cops have better access to the easiest way to kill themselves than most people. I have, with me or in my house at all times, my service weapon. But the reason it made me laugh is because Ben doesn't realize what a coward I am. I would be waaaaaaayyy too scared to ever kill myself. For one, my pain threshold is way too low. Hell, I stub my toe and I'm down for six months. Secondly, I've got too much to do before it's time to naturally check out.

But the fact that he'd thought about it and jumped in feet first to make sure it didn't happen touched me pretty good.

My doctor made me have a PET scan, which is a multi-hour test where you can't move at all and are strapped to a table and then slipped into a machine, sort of like ground sausage jammed into the casing. That test was to take a look, head to toe, and see if the cancer had spread.

It came back negative. No spread, no indication of any cancer anywhere.

The Interferon treatment I have to do is cautionary. The oncologist says let's take the drugs, do the protocol. It will soup up your immune system and make sure that if there is a handful of cancer cells anywhere in my cranky little body, they'll die a horrible, horrible death.

Hey, better them than me, right?

Comments

Nick K, Nov 27, 2005

I'm keeping good thoughts for you, Trey.

John P, Nov 27, 2005

Jeez, man, I had no idea! Thank God they didn't have to amputate your neck. That would have been awkward.

Trey to Nick K, Nov 28, 2005

Thanks so much for your thoughts, I appreciate it. I'll be fine and when this is all over we'll go have some cheap Mexican beer. Wait, maybe that's what gave me cancer...hmmmm.

Trey to John P, Nov 28, 2005

"Every head turns...except hers, she has no neck. HAHAHAHA."

Sorry, just can't not quote Steve Martin. You know, John, I had been doing just fine. No more depression, no more wondering about my mortality and shit like that. And here you come with one more itty bitty thing to worry about. Neck amputation! Hell, I'm not even sure my insurance would cover that! And wouldn't I have to get rid of my collared shirts? Wow, so many things to consider.

John P, Nov 28, 2005

On the bright side, you could say good-bye to neckties...(Seriously, I'm really glad that you're doing better.)

Jim M, Dec 4, 2005

Kick its ass, Trey. Here's hoping for a fast and complete recovery.

Part 2
November 30, 2005 – 2:09 pm

The dreams have been sort of strange.

They started the very first night after the docs told me it was malignant melanoma. I usually dream pretty vividly, but I don't usually remember everything or for very long.

I remember everything from the first night's dream.

I was in full uniform, with badge and handcuffs and weapon and extra ammunition and everything else that goes with being a cop. I was back at my high school, Robert E. Lee in Midland, Texas. We were in an auditorium, but not the one I remember from high school more than twenty years ago. This one, instead, was large but square, had only two doors, both on the same wall, no windows, and no stage doors.

A man, and I think he had a gun of some sort, had taken a pile of hostages and put himself on the wall between the two doors. The Midland Police Department was there and they wore their mid-1970's uniforms, the uniforms of my childhood.

For whatever reason, those policemen couldn't get the situation in hand. For whatever reason, they called me. And somehow, though I live twenty or twenty two hours away, I got home pretty quickly.

Because of my work in theater and because I had graduated from Lee High, I was the only one who knew there was a catwalk above the auditorium. It began over the stage, but then extended out into the house, all the way to the back of the auditorium. And though the auditorium was different from reality, the catwalk was exactly right.

Going out in the house meant it also went out over where the bad guy stood.

You see where this is going, right?

I went into the catwalk and in spite of all the gear clanking around (ever notice how loud cops are when they walk unless they're taking special care?), managed to get directly above the bad guy without him noticing. Luckily for me, there was an eight inch by eight inch hole in the catwalk.

I slipped the barrel of my Glock 21 through the hole and fired once. The bad guy looked a little surprised, then slumped to the floor and the dream dissipated.

"What's that mean?" I asked my wife.

She looked at me incredulously, like she does so often when I say something stupid, and said, "Are you serious? You can't figure that out? You don't feel like maybe you're being held hostage right now?"

Uh…yeah…that's what I meant.

In that dream, and in the others I've had since I got the diagnosis, I'm always in trouble or danger. The accoutrements are all different and don't really matter. I mean, I haven't seen a Midland cop in twenty years, I haven't visited Lee High school since 1995 and haven't been to Midland since 1997. Those little pieces, the window dressing, don't matter at all.

What matters is the jeopardy, the fact that I'm in danger. I've had a pretty good life, never had giant problems or disasters. I wasn't molested, never been shot or stabbed, never had a serious disease. Even my heart attack a few years ago was fairly mild, though it scared the shit outta me.

The cancer makes the heart attack look like a mid-afternoon respite at Johnny's Barbeque in Midland. And speaking of my favorite barbeque place, what does it say that in the very first dream, mere hours after getting the diagnosis, I dreamt I was back in my hometown, back where I grew up and always felt safe?

But what matters more to me than the danger is the fact that in all the dreams so far, I've always gotten out of it. Whether by being Supercop or an Indiana Jones style hero or whatever, I've always saved myself and gone on with life.

And I gotta say, I look pretty cool in Indy's hat.

Comments

Mom, Dec 3, 2005

I always did like you in that style of hat! And you have always killed all the bad guys in time for the commercial.

Part 3: Day One of Interferon
Monday, December 5th, 2005

Holy damn, I'm shaking.

I asked the nurse how long it would be until the chills set in. She said different times for different people. Take note: for me? About 4 1/2 seconds.

Today was the first day of chemo. While I wasn't terrified, I was certainly in the ballpark of scared. What's going to happen? How hard is it going to hit me? Will I even be able to walk when the first dose is over? Or will I be a pile of blubber in the floor, wearing my Texas boots and waiting for housekeeping to scoop me up and toss me out with the biodegradables?

(Mom always said make sure you have clean underwear and that your boots are shined...can't die with dirty boots, it's so trailer trash.)

None of those terrible things happened, at least not yet — now two hours after the first dose. But the day is still young! I could be tossing my Tex-Mex lunch cookies within in the hour.

I got there a few minutes early but had to wait for nearly an hour as I had been unable to take my medicine an hour before. It's Indomethacin, a blood thinner that helps with all manner of side effects. I can't remember exactly what right now, as I seem to be a little brain muddy, but it's a good thing, I'm told.

The RN — a woman named Jodi — tried to put in the IV needle and blew one of my veins. Hurt like hell. She popped it out and went at it again. The second time took but still hurt like hell. Then I got 100 cc's of saline and about halfway through that, the oncology nurse came in, hooked up a bag of Interferon, and off we went.

Four and a half seconds later, I was shaking with some USDA Prime Grade A Super Deluxe Double Oh Seven Can't Tell You I'd Have To Kill You chills, and it seemed like

Sorry, had to stop for a minute.

(I thought about editing out the sentence fragment, but this is what's happening and I want this journal to be as true to what's going on as it can be…just be thankful I'm fixing the spelling and typing mistakes because my fingers belong to someone else right now…maybe they belong to Tom Pic and he's toying with me like I'm a cheap voodoo doll or something…nah, not Tom.)

The shakes are getting worse, but I have no muscle pain. I'm pretty sure that'll happen but maybe not until I'm driving down the highway at 80 or 90. hehehehe…okay, not particularly funny. For those of who you thought cancer would make me funnier, sorry.

There was a slight burn at the needle when the Interferon began bubbling through the lines and into me. Not like hot burn, but sting burn. Just a touch. Just enough to make me think about it. No point to that detail, really, just interesting is all.

The nurse told me symptoms might manifest in minutes or hours, but she also said that whatever symptoms I might have probably would dissipate within six or eight hours. That would be great. That they might go away just about the time I try to go to bed is great news. I already sleep badly, tossing these symptoms on top of that might be ugly.

As I write this, the fronts of my thighs are beginning to hurt. Just a little ache, as though I had run a few hundred yards or had a really zesty bout of — Well, never mind. This is supposed to be a look at my cancer, not my libido.

Now that I take stock, I do have a few aches and pains. A bit of a thud across the top of my back, my thighs, and my calves a little.

I look back over this post and realize I haven't really said anything, just tossed a bunch of details out without any context or meaning. But I'm not sure there is any context right now. The overall context of cancer and treatment, yeah, but no snapshot context, nothing with heavy meaning or great insight into this single moment.

Maybe that's okay. Maybe the meaning is that this is simply a day in the life, simply a day where I do what needs to be done to stay alive, to make sure I am NED, with much less drama than that sentence would imply. (By the by, NED is, according to an email from a writer friend of mine who's already been through this shit, No Evidence of Disease…a good state to be in, I would think.)

I'm okay with no great meaning. Maybe less drama and more matter of fact will keep my head from getting goofy.

Getting goofy? Hah, I'll let you supply your own joke.

Part 4: Interferon Day Two
December 6, 2005 – 4:06 pm

Man, this is one funky ass ride.

While I was getting the Interferon, I thought about the journal. I thought I might start it with something like, "Second verse, same as the first," because in the first ten minutes or so, it wasn't a problem.

It was as it was last night. Day One gave me chills and a little bit of muscle pain but it was completely gone by 8:00 or 8:30. I thought, Dude this is manageable, this is doable.

"Second verse, worse than the first."

I live one block as the crow flies from the hospital and as very few people in Princeton have a fence of any kind, I just trudge through the side yard of both the auction man and the Viet vet.

Yesterday, it was a tough walk because it was 17 degrees (hello…this ain't Texas).

Today it was hard because I fucking hurt! Muscle pain, chills even worse than yesterday, hard to catch my breath. Plus it was cold…like 10 degrees or something.

The oncology nurse, name of Terre, who is waaaaaayyyyy better at stabbing me with an IV than the lady yesterday, said the side effects pile up, like NASCAR racers when someone loses it on the track rather than having the courtesy of going into the infield (or whatever they call it). This will get worse the longer I go.

Oh, goody.

Yesterday, I thought I was Batman (my favorite superhero because he's mentally damaged goods…I dig that). Today, I pretty much felt like a heroin junkie long since overdosed, with meat actually rotting off my body and the bugs already chewing on my tongue. Mmmm Mmmm Mmmm good. Can it and call me Mr. Campbell.

I plopped on the couch to watch reruns of "Star Trek: Next Generation," (yeah, I'm still a geek at heart) and it was the episode where the four ensigns are being evaluated for a secret mission. I've seen it, I know what's what, I know the young, hot blonde (even hotter than her first appearance on the show) was going to get wiped, blasted by fascist Cardassians. I knew that, knew it was coming.

And bawled like a Bon-Bon eating housefrau watching "Titanic" for the 97th time. I mean industrial grade bawlling. Tears and sloppy snot and just a touch of verbalizing.

WTF?

After the pansy-ass heart attack February 18, 2001 (RIP, Dick, have a heavenly shot for me), the meds made me much more emotional, more prone to crying at formulaic Hollywood flicks.

All right, all right, keep your comments to yourself. I'm still the acerbic, generally pissed off writer with a solid core of cynicism and emotional detachment from most of humanity. I did not change the license plate on the Mustang.

Thanks to a required two liters of water a day, I'm pissing like the outflow valve on a freakin' cruise ship and I've had my coat, and my knit cap, on now for better than two hours, trying to get warm.

Ain't working so I might well toss LuAnn out of the bed tonight and cuddle up with a space heater.

So that's where we are. Hopefully, I'll be able to write tomorrow and give you the details of Perry Memorial Hospital, Room 309. So take care and keep your knees loose.

I have no idea what that means but it's how Keith Olbermann signs off *Countdown* every night and I like how it sounds because it sounds kinda nasty…hehehehehehe.

Is my mom reading this?

Comments

Toni S, Dec 6, 2005

Just hang in there. My sister-in-law beat Leukemia. It was a very close call, but she is here now and cancer free. You sound like you have a kick-ass attitude. I'm rooting for you.

Mom, Dec 6, 2005

Yep, she is reading it. And wanting to come up there and wrap you up in a quilt and feed you chicken soup.

Trey to Mom, Dec 7, 2005

And here I was worried you'd want to come up and kick my ass for liking Olbermann's tag line so much.

Trey, in response to the descriptive tag line on a commenter's avatar, Dec 7, 2005

All hail the Queen of self-inflicted drama? That's even better than Olbermann's tag line. I love it! Might have to steal it…course I'm not really a Queen…as far as y'all know.

Seriously, thanks for the words, I appreciate them. I suspect at the next con we'll all be drinking a toast that I'm not dead. Have to figure out a way to make the hotel pay for it 'cause I sure as hell will be broke….

Part 5: Drugs and Community
December 7, 2005 – 5:16 pm

Zowie zonky…said the honky.

Sooooo much better today. Yesterday turned into a disaster. Chills that simply increased and increased, even beyond what I wrote about, until I thought my teeth would shatter. I actually did bite into my tongue twice. Good amount of muscle pain, a massive headache.

Today? Almost nothing. The chills are negligible, zero muscle pain, no headache, no snotty nose. I have no idea why the difference. I drank my two liters of water before the infusion, maybe that helped. It wasn't as cold on the walk home, maybe that made a difference. When I got home I went straight to work on my novel, the space heater on and my mind on something else. Maybe that helped.

Regardless, today was so much better…though I do find myself getting some chills right now. Maybe today wasn't better as much as postponed.

So, the nurse who had such a hard time hitting a vein the first day? Turns out she's the daughter of the nurse who did such a great job stabbing me the second day. I'm thinking Mom needs to have a sit down with daughter. "Okay, take Dad's hand, line the needle up. No, no, take it out, let's do it again. Practice makes perfect."

Room 309. Smallish room, all the bells and whistles of a standard hospital room. But there is an interesting painting by a Bernard Buffet. French guy. The painting is called something like "Somme River" something. It's a French village with the River Somme running through the middle of it. Lots of scratches and slices in the oranges and yellows. Elongated splashes in the middle of the sky and the river. I've no idea what style it is, but it's cool. A little too symmetrical for my taste but not bad for an institution.

The room is right above the ambulance bay so every time a bus comes in, sirens blaring, I hear it. Actually heard the EMTs today. Sounded pretty stressed out. Hopefully they didn't have to call the coroner a few minutes later.

Not much to say today because it went so well. Does that mean it will all be well? Or does that simply mean the Interferon gods chose to screw with me a little? "Hey, since he's sure it's going to be bad, let's give him a good day, then we'll sock the hell out of him Thursday."

We'll see. Maybe I can sacrifice a virgin to the gods and get them to leave me alone for the entire run. Of course, I'd have to know a virgin first....

***

An amazing thing happened when I told a couple of people what was going on: every one in my writing community — horror and crime — knew about it within hours.

I began getting emails and phone calls and damn near smoke signals from so many of the writers and fans and editors I'd known for so long, and quite a few emails from people I've never met, people with whom I've never corresponded.

That really freaked me out.

Everyone had positive things to say and quite a few offered to send me their latest projects to read since I'll have a bit of downtime. Everyone wished me the best.

It was really touching. I don't normally care for sentimentality, it drives me bugfuck; sugary bullshit that means squat and is nothing more than a societal obligation. But this was amazing. Everyone seemed genuinely concerned.

And everyone had a story. Their mother or father or daughter or cousin or whoever had been hit with the cancer stick and all of them survived; five years, ten years, seventeen years in one case.

Yeah, the emails are great for my ego but it goes deeper than that. I realize I'm not the first to suffer this kind of thing, but when I got hit with it, I felt pretty alone. Yeah, yeah, they've all known someone with cancer, but until you've been through it, you don't really know, not deep down, not where the scary details pile up until you can barely breathe.

They don't know, but that didn't stop them from saying, "Anything you need, you tell me and I'm right there."

And then something very cool happened. Three writers I admire greatly got in touch. They had been through it, they knew exactly. They understood everything. They knew the trepidation of that first day of chemo. They understood being concerned about the depression and wondering if this pain or that ache meant anything.

I like to consider myself quite the loner. The Texas boy who drinks whiskey straight up, wears boots and loud, colorful shirts, reads obscure writers and watches independent flicks so that I can sound more intellectual than the average rodent. What this proved to me was that, for all that posturing and public persona building (even if it is mostly the real me), they didn't care.

The arguments with some of them about how their latest project was crap, the yelling matches about how this or that bestselling writer was nothing but a half-wit; none of that meant anything. Set that aside, they basically said, because we've got this other thing to deal with.

Then, when you're healthy again, we'll kick your ass and throw your shot of Daniel's in your face.

I love this community of writers and fans and editors and publishers way more than I thought.

Maybe I'm not quite the loner I thought I was.

Damn.

Comments

Diorling, Dec 8, 2005

This one time, at band camp... (j/k). My great grandmother had to have a mastectomy, and she lived to be 83. My grandmother, currently 82 and cancer free after having breast cancer the first time in her very early 60's and NOT doing the chemo, then it came back, but in her lyph nodes (the kiss of death, usually)...so she did the chemo. It sucked, as you well know.

When the doctor interviewed her for reconstructive surgery, he peered at her little A cup 70+ year old bra and said, "Ya know...while we're in there...we could make them BIGGER." Her little eyes brightened, and she said, "Why, thank you. I think I'll have a B." And so she did...and wore them proudly.

Part 6
December 11, 2005 – 12:35 pm

I gotta tell you, I'm feeling a little gypped.

I mean, I was promised all these side effects and for the most part, I'm getting squat.

Don't get me wrong, I'll take it. The fewer side effects the better. The thing is, everyday I get psyched up for the crap and for the most part it doesn't happen. You know what that means, right? About mid week during week two, I'll stop getting psyched up for it and every single side effect known to man will hit me as hard as drunks hit my jail booking room floor when they finally pass out.

With the exception of Tuesday and Friday night, the first week of chemo was decent. A few chills, a couple of headaches, no big problem. Friday night, however, I had a massive dizzy spell that left me sitting in the middle of the floor at a local pharmacy.

I had skipped dinner because the thought of pizza made me want to yak up everything I've eaten since 1978. But at the same time, I was jonesing like a heroin fiend for Gummi Bears.

Yeah, yeah, I know, Gummi Bears. One of the more macho foods out there.

So I went to a pharmacy that happens to have Gummis along with all the drugs you could ever want and snapped up two bags. I was standing at the front counter, talking to Lisa the pharmacist, when she looked at me askance and asked if I was okay, did I want to sit down.

"Nah, I'm fine," I said, full of macho manliness, a bag of Gummis in each tight little fist.

Two seconds later, I was on the floor. And remember, I was at her counter…where customers with snow on their shoes had been standing all day.

Yeah, wet ass, dizzy head, cold chills…and I dropped my Gummi Bears (oh, the final indignity!).

Managed to drive home (I know, not particularly bright but there it is) and went straight to bed…dreamt of Gummis all night long.

Of the few side effects I am having, one of the more interesting is what it's doing to my sense of taste. The nurse said I would get to where steak tasted metallic and greasy fast food — the most healthy of all foods — would make me gag.

So far, though only one thing tastes like crap.

Coca Cola.

AAAAAAAaaaaaaauuuugggg!!!!

Coke? Had to be Coke, right? Couldn't be green beans or beets or whatever. Had to be Coke. 'Course, I guess there is an argument to be made that green beans and beets already taste like crap…at least to me.

I've not tried Dr Pepper yet since I started the Interferon so I don't know if the Elixir from the Sacred Homeland (Dr Pepper and I are both from Texas…like that means anything to anyone except…well…me) sucks, too.

So one week in, my complaints are fairly mild. I realize I've got it pretty good so far, better than so many other people. I'm not throwing up, I'm not losing my hair, I'm not spending twenty-three hours a day in bed, I'm not hoping the radiation kills the cancer before it kills me.

I know it's cumulative, I know it'll get worse. I just hope my jokes will still be funny when I'm really sick.

Comments

Toni S, Dec 11, 2005

I love your sense of humor. It will help you get through this. Just take it one day at a time.

T.J. C, Dec 11, 2005

The curative powers of Dr Pepper are not to be underestimated.

Part 7
December 14, 2005 – 9:21 am

The metaphor is too easy.

It's been snowing since just before my first Interferon treatment. Cold and snowy and overcast and sunless and whatever else you want to say.

The metaphor is too easy.

Last time I wrote, I mentioned I was feeling a little ripped off. Hah, no more. Monday and Tuesday were more along the lines of what I expected. Last Friday, I had a bit of dizziness and light headedness (I know, I know, how can you tell?). Same thing happened Monday and Tuesday after the treatments.

Monday night wasn't horrible, just enough to get my attention. But Tuesday, even the nurses at Perry Memorial noticed something. They made me sit for a while after the treatment. Eventually I felt okay and walked on home (I'm about a block from the hospital, no big deal).

An hour after I got home, one of the deputies called to check on me. As I hung up from that phone call, it all came up. Dizzy. Light headed. Suddenly exhausted. Headache. And, for nearly five full, loverly minutes, industrial strength vomiting.

Welcome to side effect land. Or rather, Side-Effectland.

For the last few days, the thought of food has not sat well with me, even though at the same time I crave all kinds of things. Aside from the Gummi craving, I've also craved McDonald's Quarter Pounder, the local Pizza Hut salad bar, and Dr Pepper.

And the Pepper, by the by, does taste like shit. Damn, my treatment is even interfering with the Elixir of Life from the Sacred Homeland.

So I try to eat mostly bland foods because I haven't quite yet figured out what makes me sick and what doesn't. A writer friend of mine said stay away from hot foods. Good advice, I'm sure, but the thought of a cold Quarter Pounder cracks me up and grosses me out.

And Holy Cripes, can I sleep anymore? Hour after hour upon hour, filled with all kinds of bizarre dreams that don't seem to have any particular through-line or plot line or metaphor anymore. No more SuperCop or Indiana Jones, no more watching planes fall out of the sky and calling 911, no more of anything around which I can decipher a relationship to what's happening in my life.

My guess is the treatments have turned my subconscious to mush, God knows it has my conscious. In fact, I've been so brain muddy that yesterday LuAnn was trying to explain something about email to me and I simply couldn't understand what she was saying. Turned out to be incredibly simple but I just couldn't get my head around it.

Makes me suddenly understand why Sgt. Atkinson, the one so worried about me when I got the diagnosis, has lately taken to calling me retard.

I know, very un-p.c., but funny. Isn't it sad how, when it's just friends, all the pc and societal politeness and all that goes straight out the fuggin' window?

Still and all, even with everything, it isn't what I expected. I expected more of everything and more things. I expected more muscle ache and more headaches. I expected hair loss and maybe a nose bleed. I expected to feel more sick more often.

I expected more of a snow storm, that the internal would more closely match the external.

I should just count it good I'm doing well enough, I guess. And the downtime has given me a ton of time for reading. And thinking about new projects, though I haven't really been able to get any decent writing done.

It's hard to tell, when I look out the window, if it's still snowing or simply blowing. I guess it doesn't really matter. As long as I can't see the street or the house next door, the cause doesn't really matter.

I'll tell you what, though, regardless of the internal, I'm getting sick and tired of all the snow. I need one good day of sunshine.

Comments

Diorling, Dec 14, 2005
   Nina Simone, "Lilac Wine."

Mom, Dec 14, 2005
   Yep, "chemo brain" is setting in. Going to be bad news for the writing for a while. Maybe all those weird dreams will eventually coalesce into The Great American Novel.

Morbidmom04, Dec 15, 2005
   Hi Trey. I'm here courtesy of T.J. C. I wish I had something intelligent to say, but this turns out to be it: Best wishes from Morbid Curiosity. I hope the chemo does its job quickly and gives you space to write, too.

Part 7.5: Being Petty
December 14, 2005 – 9:46 am

I don't have treatments on Saturday or Sunday. A small respite from the needles and wondering what kinds of side effects I'll have that day.

So Saturday, I took the train to Chicago for a book signing I had scheduled long ago. The signing went fine except I was too tired to really get into it. But I got to spend some time with Jay Bonansinga, one of the absolute gentlemen in the business.

I climbed on the train in Princeton, *sans* ticket. I almost never pre-purchase a ticket, I just get it on the train. Never had a problem. This particular day, one of the conductors starts giving me static about if the train fills up with people who have reservations, I'll have to stand.

"What? I've never heard of that before," I said, more than a little surprised.

"Policy. If everyone else has a reservation and you don't, you have to stand." A sneering little voice, full of the power of being conductor.

"Not a problem," I said (and to be honest, I'm sure I had copped an attitude). "But I've been taking cancer treatments and sometimes they make me a little weak. So if we can work around the fact that I might fall over, that's not a problem."

"Should have gotten a reservation, then, huh?" he said. Then he glared at me and asked for a picture ID.

I didn't give him my license. I didn't give him either my Colorado or Illinois ID card.

I gave him my Bureau County Sheriff's Office ID card.

Hah, suck on that, bub.

There was at least thirty seconds of dead silence. He just stared and stared, then cleared his throat, finished selling me a ticket, and walked off.

I never heard another word out of him until the end of the ride. When I was getting the box of books I had taken with me, he said, "Do you need any help with that, sir?"

I am so freakin' petty. Of course I handed him the Sheriff's card hoping he'd get intimidated and leave me alone. Of course I wanted to wipe the smug grin off his face. Screw with me? I grew up in Texas, I know how to be a petty lawman don't think I don't.

Oh, and remember this: the car never filled up. The seat next to me never got taken.

Comments

Noivad, Dec 14, 2005

You had a jerk and handled it well. Not only did you put him in his place, you did it gracefully. More power to you.

Thomas R, Dec 14, 2005

Dude....one piece of good news and one piece of bad news, courtesy of T.J. C.....I don't know what to say, so I should just shut the fuck up, but of course I won't, 'cause I can't resist telling you that you're a bad ass and cancer should tremble in its friggin' boots.

Tribe, Dec 14, 2005

The previous comment reminds of a story (likely apocryphal) that I heard right after Johnny Cash died. The story goes that Johnny was sitting looking out the window a few days before he had to go to the hospital. Supposedly a buzzard takes perch in a tree outside the window, and stares at the Man In Black, who in turn stares right back at the buzzard until the buzzard gives up and flies away.

The story is likely bullshit...but it should be true.

Toni S, Dec 16, 2005

    The feel of sweet satisfaction when you kick someone's ass without really lifting a finger is nice, ain't it?

Part 8
Monday, December 19th, 2005

Everything, except milk and orange sherbet, tastes like shit.

But I think I'm getting a handle on this whole food thing (as opposed to a whole foods thing). Usually, I can eat most things for about ten or fifteen minutes before whatever it is starts tasting like ass. I'm assuming, from all my years in medical school, that it takes about that long for the Interferon to seep back out through my taste buds and coat everything I eat.

I've noticed, too, that if I have some water before I eat, I can usually get through the entire meal without the food tasting bad. Maybe the water acts as a cleanser, I have no idea.

But, even if I know how to make it taste decently, most times the mere thought of food makes me want to holler. I've eaten mostly nothing but salads for two weeks and while I like the weight I'm losing, I wouldn't recommend this particular diet plan to those of you looking to shed those unsightly holiday pounds.

And I can't tell you how tired I am of water. Holy cripes. Two liters a day and it's mostly water because everything else tastes bad. Coke. Dr Pepper. Gatorade. Fruit punch. Whatever.

The last few days weren't terrible for side effects with the exception of being light headed and muddy brained. Friday, Saturday, and a few minutes on Sunday saw me at the edge of passing out at odd, random moments. I get overheated very easily and then woozy and dizzy and the rest.

The muddy brained? There seems to be nothing in particular that sets that off, it's just a general state right now. Sucks, though, because I can't remember anything and sometimes have a hard time putting together a sentence.

Actually, I think it might be an interesting, decidedly superficial, look at the beginnings of the dementia you know I'm going to get when I get old.

I've been thinking about 'why me' this weekend; you know, along the lines of "Why did this horrible thing happen to me?" I haven't come to any conclusions, though I did finally decide the question did not pre-suppose any sort of God or Gods.

Really, though, the entire question is fairly ego-centric, ain't it? Why me basically asks why something in the universe thought me worthy of the cancer stick.

I think I probably think it's random. Just like the drunk that barrels through an intersection and kills four kids on their way to soccer practice while barely getting a scratch, or why a string of six numbers comes up on the very day a 98-year old woman bought a Lottery ticket with those six numbers.

Andy Dufrense has a line in *Shadwshank Redemption* that's good right now. He and Red are talking about bad luck. He says something like "It's gotta land on somebody, I guess it was just my turn."

And let's be clear: I don't consider myself in the same league as people undergoing radiation treatment or who've had debilitating strokes or whose four kids were just killed by that drunk. My situation is not anywhere near as dire as theirs, but it is my situation and it does seem pretty bad in my relative terms.

I'm at the halfway point. Two more weeks of the daily treatments, then eleven months of the self-injections. Also, in a couple of weeks, assuming no disasters, I can go back to work. I haven't really missed work yet. That is to say, I don't really miss fighting with drunks. Laughing at those drunks as they stumble around and ask me why they were arrested, yeah, I miss that but only because I'm mean and petty.

But then, we all knew that, didn't we?

Part 9
December 21, 2005 – 10:33 am

Yeah, the men and women at the sheriff's office are sooooooo supportive and helpful.

Knowing I can't hardly eat, this is the call I get this morning.

"Hey, how about a greasy hamburger?"

In the back ground, "And the greasy fries, too."

"Yeah, and some greasy fries and a big ol' Dr Pepper?"

In the background, "I get off at 11, I'll bring him some Gummi Bears."

And then a barrage of laughter that boomed through the phone like a friggin' explosion.

Yeah, thanks so much for all that, you guys. Nothing like support from your co-workers. Just hearing them ask me about greasy food almost made me throw-up.

And yet, there is still a part of me craving exactly those things. How perverse is that? To crave what you know will make you sick.

Food and fatigue, those are the things. Most food tastes awful but even if it tasted good, I've got no appetite. And I'm sleeping the better part of 15 to 18 hours a day. When I'm awake, I'm weak, hardly able to walk up the stairs and even drag my ass to the bathroom to spit out a mouthful of white nastiness that, I suppose, is the Interferon.

This week, the third week of four, has so far been much rougher than the first two. I had thought I was getting robbed during the first weeks; lots of talk about side effects, but really none to speak of.

Actually, now that I think about it, didn't I write about this yesterday? OR maybe the day before. When ever.

Two new things. The first is that I'm having a hard time walking home from the hospital. It's about a block and a half from my house and this week, that block is tough (though, again, my co workers came to my rescue. One of the deputies said, "Hell, I've crawled further than that getting home from a bar!").

Yesterday I called Ben Atkinson, my friend of retard fame, and asked if he could drive me home. He shows up, gets me home, and then sits in the driveway, watching me until I get damn near to the door.

"Wanna make sure you don't get jiggy in the snow," he called from the warmth of his car.

Jiggy in the snow? Ain't that a dance or something?

Cancer: got a good beat, I can get jiggy in the snow to it. I give it a 98.

Speaking of 98, I've had a fever most of the week. Standing in 17 degree weather wanting to do nothing so much as strip to the skin and get jiggy (or jiggly, whichever).

The main new thing is the anger. I find I'm pissed all the time. Not like early on, when I joked about being mad at the whole concept of cancer. Now I'm furious. I don't want to deal with this bullshit.

I hate the disease, I hate the treatment. I hate the nurses and the stupid-ass painting in the room. I hate the perfume one of the nurses wears, a perfume I'll never be able to smell again without thinking of all this crap.

I have to leave earlier and earlier to get to the hospital because I walk so much more slowly than I did. I don't understand the why or the fairness or any of the rest of it. I'm bored outta my fucking skull (at least during those rare and short stretches when I'm not asleep), and I am so weak I can't even hardly hold a book!

I hate everything about this bullshit. What else is there to say?

Comments

Toni S, Dec 21, 2005

And this too shall pass. I hate to hear that you don't have better support, by support, I mean someone there with you. Listen to music, music like Mozart. Good and peaceful.

Also, you need to get some of those Ensure nutritional shakes. Try to drink those, even if they taste like crap. You are so tired partially because you are not getting the nutrients you need through your diet.

And it's okay to be mad. I don't blame you. Repressing that anger will not help. If someone pisses you off, tell them to fuck off. Tell them why you are mad. Your co-workers probably think they are cheering you up, joking around with you. Tell them what they can do to help.

People get nervous when someone is really sick. They don't know what to do to help and they often say the wrong things or do the wrong things in their feeble attempts at maintaining the normalcy. This is your life. Don't let anyone else add anymore misery to it. Keep your chin up above the water and keep on swimming. *hugs*

Part 10: Of The Psychology
Wednesday, December 28th, 2005

I think there is an interesting psychological element going on.

The side effects have generally gotten worse as time slips past, but this week — week four of four — hasn't been terrible. There have been days when I was utterly exhausted, but there have also been days when I got up in the morning feeling pretty damned good. And quite a bit of the anger is gone.

Why, I wonder, when the dosage is the same and there is more medicine built up down in my guts, do I seem to be doing better?

Is it because I know I'm almost done? Today is Wednesday and Friday is the last daily treatment. Could it be that knowing I'm almost done makes everything a little brighter? And let's not discount the weather, either. The first three weeks were bitterly cold. Last few days have been beautiful. Cold but only in the 30s rather than single digits.

There are a ton of people coming by the house or stopping at the hospital to pick me up and maybe that's helping, too. They've started to check in with me more often, I think, because they knew the treatments were getting so harsh last week.

Maybe all of that together is what's helping, I don't know. But I do know this week hasn't been as bad as I thought it was going to be.

I'm still tired. And everything still sucks when it comes to food.

But I seem to have a better outlook.

I don't know yet when I'll go back to work, hopefully next week. I think part of the problem was looking ahead to four weeks of doing nothing. I had hoped to get some writing done, work on some initial thoughts for a new series character, finish up a few short stories.

I did squat. No writing. No reading. I didn't even work on my sudoku puzzles, which I'm all kinds of goofy about.

But I do see a light at the end of the tunnel and that's good. Then we'll start phase II: self injections. I have no idea what that'll be like yet but it can't be any worse than what I've been through.

So, I'm taking a breath, taking a walk, counting down the days...sort of like a cancer-ridden Dick Clark counting down his big ball on New Year's.

Part 11: The End of the Beginning
January 2, 2006 – 1:22 pm

Friday was my birthday.

Friday was also the last day of daily Interferon treatments.

Not quite the birthday I had planned but given the context, not bad at all. Hey, no more going to the hospital every day, no more getting stabbed (my hands look like friggin' pin cushions from all the IVs), no more of the one nurse's perfume.

No more of any of that crap.

I consider this the end of the first part of all this bullshit; of initial tests and surgery and what a writer friend of mine called Interferon Boot Camp, and all the rest of the bullshit that goes with being a stage 3 cancer survivor (and how odd is it to think that about yourself?).

Now we move on to the thrice weekly injections (from now until December, 2006) and I have no idea what that means. Will I be as tired, sleeping 15 hours a day? Will I be able to eat anything? Will I be as cranky and pissed as I have been?

It's the same medicine but only three times a week rather than five, and a smaller dosage. I suspect I'll begin to feel somewhat normal again.

On the other hand, even today (Monday, four days since my last treatment) lunch still tasted like crap. Of course, it was week old Hamburger Helper so maybe that had more to do with the food than the medicine.

It is entirely possible I'll have all the same side effects for the next year. It's possible they'll be less than they are now, but it's also possible they'll be just as bad.

Yeah, can you see me at the jail, feeling tired and hardly able to walk, just as a drunk who likes to fight gets arrested?

"Uh, excuse me, sir, I'm kind of tired, can you wait to fight until the next shift? I'd appreciate it."

I don't think it'll be that bad. I think I'll feel much closer to my old cynical self than I do now...though I suspect it'll be next Christmas before I feel completely normal.

Here's an odd tidbit about the injections. It might be more expensive to do it myself. Yeah, welcome to modern American insurance bullshit. More expensive to do it at home than it would be to go do it at the hospital, where I'd have to take up a nurse's time, use an ambulatory services room, labs and registration, all the rest of it.

WTF? And insurance companies wonder why people hate them.

Last week, the oncology nurse began working on how I'd get the injections. We don't know yet because the insurance company hasn't returned any calls. In other words, yeah, they'll take my money every month but won't pick up a damned phone.

In the middle of everything I've been through in the last six weeks, here is the thought that makes me the craziest: I'll never know if the treatment worked.

Thousands and thousands of dollars and it's basically to prove a negative. Regardless of the treatment, the cancer might come back (do I get my money back if that happens?). Or it might never come back because the surgery got it all. I have no idea.

I want to say — as publicly as I can — thanks to two writers who have been absolutely incredible during the last six weeks. You've heard of both of them and you've read their books and stories, and both of them are either currently fighting cancer or are currently in remission. Without them, I'm not sure I could have done as well as I have. I realized in the last few days how much I love both of them...for things I'll probably never be able to tell them.

(Hah, how funny is this? Isreal Kamakawewo'ole's version of "Somewhere Over the Rainbow" is playing right now on the bookstore stereo.)

Comments

George (Sleepless in Midland Blog), Jan 2, 2006

Happy Birthday!

And man oh man! I sure do hope you pull through this thing in fine shape.

Scanner_Darkly, Jan 2, 2006

You know, I always want to post something, and I never know what to say. "Wow, that's really messed up" seems so...trivial, but it's all I got.

Hang in there, ok?

Aldo, Jan 3, 2006

Happy Birthday!

This is a new year and new beginnings. Tina and I have in you in our thoughts and prayers. Things can only look upwards from here.

All the best.

Toni S, Jan 3, 2006

Happy belated birthday.

Now maybe you can get this stuff behind you and focus on enjoying life instead of just trying to keep your head above the dark water.

Ellen D, Jan 4, 2006

Happy Birthday, Trey – and many more. Mine was Saturday

Rick and Julie T, Jan 6, 2006

happy belated birthday trey...wish i knew i could have had somebody come dance for u!!!

....miss your face and am still saying those prayers.....
just me and Julie

Trey to Rick and Julie T, Jan 6, 2006
     If you come dance for me, I want you wearing nothing
but the gun belt, the badge, and those sexy cop boots, you big,
burly he-man of a guy.

Trey to Ellen D, Jan 6, 2006
     Happy Birthday, Ellen. I hope all is well with you,
knowwhadda mean?

Ellen D, Jan 6, 2006
     Yup. thanks

Trey to Scanner Darkly, Jan 6, 2006
     It's more than enough. Just the thought does me good.
     Thank you.

Trey to Aldo, Jan 6, 2006
     Thanks so much, Aldo.
     Things are already looking up. See the next installment of
Cancer Chronicles, written sometime in the next twenty minutes
or so.

Trey to George, Jan 6, 2006
     George! Been a while. Thanks so much for the good
wishes and keep up the brilliant work on Sleepless in Midland.

Trey to Toni S, Jan 6, 2006
     Enjoying life? Perish the thought! Seriously, thanks for all
your good wishes over the last weeks, I do appreciate them. And
yeah, I'm enjoying things more now than in the recent past...and
getting outta the damned house has been a major part of that.

Part 12: Life Starts at 39
January 6, 2006 – 6:24 pm

Holy guacamole! It's all so different.

Friday, Dec. 30 was the last of the heavy duty treatments.

Tuesday, Jan 3, was the first of the easier treatments. I went from an hour a day, five days a week in the hospital getting about fifty gallons of Interferon to three times a week getting something like 20 milli-somethings.

It's great but the best news first.

Dr Pepper is beginning to taste good again. Not always and not completely, but it's getting there. And there are all kinds of foods I can eat again. Hah, the challenge now will be to not gorge myself on friggin' hamburgers and fries and garbage so that I can keep the twenty pounds off.

Tuesday I went back to the hospital, my stomach in knots because I had no clue what was going to happen, how the injection portion of all this was going to work. The nurses, as they had been for four weeks previous, were fabulous. They seemed to have learned how to read me, how to know when I wanted to gab and when I was surly and needed silence.

The shot came in a syringe with an incredibly fine needle. It was like hair, and when she pinched up a bit of my abdomen and jammed the needle in, I felt absolutely nothing.

And for those of you who know me a bit, you know how incredible that is. I am a complete lunatic about needles. Show me a needle and I might well start to cry. Shit, the inmates in my jail ever figure that out and I'm screwed.

It took me longer to ride the elevator up to the third floor than it did to get the shot.

I was a little tired afterward, but not much. I went to work to talk with my boss about getting back on the schedule, talked to a few others, laughed a lot — almost giddily because I couldn't believe I wasn't having any problems.

And promptly threw up.

I'd only done that once before during the treatments and it was quite the little surprise. But I hosed myself. I have meds that will take care of the nausea and I didn't bother taking them, thinking the shot wouldn't be a problem.

Then I fell asleep for about five days.

Uh…okay, maybe the shot's a little tougher on me than I thought it would be.

But still so much better. I'm pretty sure I'll have the same side effects, but to a lesser degree.

Hell, as long as Dr Pepper tastes good again, I'll take the rest. Yeah, there's a priority. Not health, not white blood cell count, not nausea…Dr Pepper.

Thursday, I had another shot — this one with a fucking 14 inch needle that was about four inches in diameter. The nurse jabbed me like a kid jabbing at found roadkill and three days later I still feel it.

I went to work right after the shot and had to drive three inmates to Stateville Prison in Joliet (remember the Blues Brothers movie? That prison.). I did pretty well most of that trip (the other deputy drove just in case I passed out or something).

We stopped for lunch on the way back and while I was able to eat, I did get fairly dizzy. No throwing up or anything. I just swallowed some Tylenol and was fine a while later.

So I'm still not sure exactly how the shots are going to go, but today I feel more like myself than I have since before the surgery that got all this started the first week of November.

I'm 39 years old now, as of last Friday, and while it doesn't feel like I've started a new chapter or dodged a bullet or gotten a new lease on life or any of the other sappy cliches, I do feel like I can stop looking backward or sideways or whatever. I got through the harshest part of all this and I'm back at work, back to writing, back to having fun with my wife.

All in all, not a bad place to be.

Comments

Stace J, Jan 6, 2006

Hi Trey,

Happy birthday. I'm still older than you, you know. I'm glad the new year is starting out well for you; I hope it continues in this … ahem … vein.

Toni S, Jan 7, 2006

It sounds like the worst is over. I hope so. It's good to hear you upbeat and not downbeat.

Ellen D, Jan 7, 2006

Trey,

Great to hear the news – especially about the old taste buds. That's important.

Part 12.5: Kissing the Angels
January 7, 2006 – 12:48 pm

A few days ago, Bureau County Judge Scott Madson asked me if I'd kissed the angels.

"What?" I asked, puzzled.

"LuAnn told me what was going on," he said.

Ah yes, the cancer, the giant white hippo hanging out on my shoulder.

In other words, did I think I was going to die?

Tough question...one that has come up before.

On Valentine's Day, February 14, 2001, my friend writer Richard Laymon died of a heart attack. Four days later, while racing back and forth between three different theater gigs in Denver, I had a heart attack.

Aside from the pain, the only thing I thought about was Dick. He was why I called 911 as quickly as I did. I spent 24 hours in cardiac ICU and the next five or six weeks recovering at home.

A month later, I went to the World Horror Convention in Seattle. Amidst the well wishes from writer friends and memorials for Dick, one publisher sat me down and asked, "So, was this a publicity stunt?"

Yeah, let me show you the picture of the cardiac before and after. Yeah, because I've made so much money, gotten so much press, from having a heart attack. What an ass. He followed that up with, "Did you think you were going to die?"

There are quite a few things that scare me, but death hasn't yet been one of those things.

In neither case, the heart attack nor the cancer, did I think I was about to cash it in. In neither case did I cozy up to any angels and give them a big wet smack on the lips.

That's not to say there weren't days when I wasn't terrified. During the 'cardiac event,' which is what the doctors called the heart attack, I was quite scared. On the ground in front of Denver's Temple Events Center, listening to the siren and knowing it tolled for me was enough to get some juices flowing. In the cardiac ICU, listening to someone a few beds down flatline was more than enough to give me a jolt.

Hearing my doctor calmly say the lump was malignant and then say stage 3 was enough to keep me awake at night. During the days between the diagnosis and the results of the PET scan I had a talk with LuAnn about the logistics of death, what to do with any literary work I had unfinished or unsold, that I wanted to be cremated, where to scatter the ashes, no machines to keep me alive, etc. We talked about death, but the conversation was somehow more obligatory than necessary.

Not once in either case did I think I was going to die. The question is: does that matter? Could I have died even though the thought that I might die never really took hold?

Obviously, yes.

But it felt to me, back in 2001 and four weeks ago, that I wouldn't die because I didn't think I would. And I'm not talking about positive mental attitude kind of bullshit. I'm talking about absolute certainty, the kind of certainty that doesn't even allow you to question where the sun will rise tomorrow morning.

Yeah, the sun rises in the east. Naw, this won't kill me.

Which leaves me with an obvious flipside, doesn't it? What happens when I have some medical problem and do see an angel or two coming at me, lips all smacked up and raring to go?

Hell, who am I kidding, it probably won't be an angel at all.

Comments

Lonesome Crow, Jan 7, 2006

Someone had the temerity to ask if your heart attack was a publicity stunt!? Sorry, but WTF!? I'm enjoying your "Cancer Chronicles." I'm quite sure you won't be cozying up to any angels soon.

Best Wishes!

Toni S, Jan 8, 2006

Wow, cancer & a heart attack? Almost sounds like a conspiracy, like the universe is trying to take you out. You must be a pretty strong guy to survive both events. Either that or someone's got your back.

Part 13
Monday, January 16th, 2006

So I think I've got a handle on the shots.

After a couple of weeks of getting them, I see a pattern.

Tuesday, Thursday, Saturday are the days, usually mid-morning. About four hours after the shot, I get incredibly light-headed for about two hours. Once that goes away, I'm simply tired for the rest of the day.

The freaky thing is that the light-headed happens so regularly I can damn near set my watch by it. I assume it's my body reacting to the new batch of medicine.

Last Saturday, I mentioned the light-headedness to one of the nurses. She said my blood pressure tends to run low right now as a matter of course, and wondered if, during the dizzy spells, it was running even lower.

"Anybody at the jail who can take your blood pressure when you get dizzy?"

Uh...yeah, all kinds of inmates...they all have some medical experience.

Actually, I kept the smart ass answer to myself and enlisted the help of a deputy who also works a local ambulance service.

Holy crap. At the hospital, my pressure was lower than normal but not much. I can't remember exactly. But during my dizzy phase, it was 89 over 63 or something.

Uh, yeah, maybe that's why I get so dizzy. Hmmmm...could be a causal relationship there.

So that's what's going on medically. No more throwing up so far, but lots of dizzy and tired. I'm getting tired of being tired all the time. Yeah, it's less than during the daily treatments, but it's still there. Rarely do I feel 100 percent like my old self.

Mostly there is a tinge of fatigue around the edges of everything I do.

And guess what? Dr Pepper taste like crap again. Actually, all soda does. Where it had been salty, now it's bitter. It doesn't matter what kind of soda, it's all bitter. I assume that has to do with the CO_2, which is the only thing they all have in common. So that sucks, although it is keeping me from drinking lots of heavily sugar laden drinks so that's probably good.

It's been good to get back to work. We've been full up but don't have any problem inmates right now so I haven't had to worry about fights or discipline or whatever. But simply getting out of this house where I've been cooped up, to get back to the people I work with (most of whom I actually dig pretty well), to get outside and remember the larger world outside my door, has been great. I think it's probably done more for my outlook than anything else.

During the daily treatments, I tried to keep up with the journal. Every day or every other day or whatever. But with the shots, there isn't as much going on. And the side effects don't build like they did. So there probably won't be as much to write about cancer wise.

Which is odd, when I think about it. Have I become so inured to this bullshit of the last two months that I have nothing left to say about it?

Back in 2000, I found out I had a half-sister. For months after that discovery, the words 'my sister' felt really odd in my mouth. It was the same way at the first diagnosis. 'Cancer,' when applied to me, was just strange.

Now it seems normal. Writer. Deputy. Cynic. Cancer.

It all fits as though that's the natural state of my life, and that fucking sucks.

Part 14
January 22, 2006 – 1:08 pm

I might have died.

On the other hand, I know my imagination sometimes gets overheated. Maybe that's as far as it would have gone.

Zip, bango, and I'm light-headed – or in what would be a blood sugar crisis for a diabetic — at 75 miles an hour and the car crashes. Flips, explodes, tosses me out like an unconscious ragdoll and suddenly LuAnn is collecting life insurance.

Saturday morning I had a treatment, about 10:00. I also had a signing scheduled at the Bloomington, IL Barnes and Noble for 3 p.m. I wasn't worried about side effects from the treatment because they've been so mild and so predictable. And they seemed to be getting better. Thursday's treatment made me light-headed — as usual — but not until six hours later and then only for an hour.

Great news. A huge step forward.

By a bit after 11 a.m. Saturday, I was light-headed. I stopped at my wife's bookstore to steal her car to take to Bloomington and when her eyes got big and scared from seeing me, I knew there was a problem.

I crashed on the little couch for about an hour and felt a little better. I was preparing to hit the road when Sgt. Atkinson came in. I thought, cool, haven't seen him in a few days, I'll talk for a minute, then leave.

I sat back on the couch and watched Ben get more and more concerned. Then LuAnn came over and started talking to me. I had no fucking clue what she was saying. Her mouth flapped and flapped, spitting something out, but I had no clue. It was creepily like when she'd tried to explain email to me in early December. I couldn't understand then, either.

It was then I decided I was good to go get some water. Hah. Nice try.

Five, maybe seven feet and I found myself staring at the shelf of Harry Potter and Unfortunate Events. From beneath it.

Ben's standing over me, white with fear because he'd never seen an actual event before. His jaw is flapping and flapping and once more I had no clue. Very odd sensation, that. Like waking up one day and everyone in your family is speaking Gaelic or maybe Sudanese.

I called and cancelled the signing while LuAnn kept freaking Ben out by saying, "Don't worry, he'll be fine, this happens all the time."

After a while, it was better. I could hear, I could understand. Ben and I went to eat — I thought that might help, it didn't — and then he drove me straight to the hospital.

Tamara, the nurse, worked me over for a few minutes, told me to drink LOTS more fluids and to get some sleep, and suddenly, I was back in the middle of December. I was back on the daily treatments with all the side effects. I was just as angry, just as whiny, as I had been in December.

I drank. I slept. (And I dreamed of being back in high school, unable to complete some stupid class assignment. Yeah, that dream actually comes along relatively regularly. We'll analyze the insecurity of that later.)

Today I'm still tired but my head is as good as ever (ha...you can supply your own joke there).

So even though Ben revels in calling me retard when I get foggy, he might well have saved my life yesterday. Had he not come in, I probably would have been on the road when the light-headedness hit. I would have been on the outskirts of the county, entombed in a single car roll-over.

And you know my co-workers would have worked the accident and radioed the sheriff, "Hey, we can use badge number 30 again, I'm pretty sure he's cashed it in."

Comments

Mom, Jan 22, 2006

Sure is scary stuff for your mom to read. But I get even more scared when you *don't* tell me what's going on. Go figure – it's a mom thing. Sounds like you better hire a limo, Mr. Big Time Writer.

Toni S, Jan 22, 2006

Glad you didn't make that trip. Be careful.

Morbid Mom, Jan 23, 2006

Yikes! I hope you are coming to the end of these treatments soon. Thanks again for telling the tale.

Dani D, Jan 30, 2006

Trey Barker who played the drums and hung out with Brad?

Dani D, Jan 30, 2006

I just read your biography and it confirms my suspicions that yes, it is you. I will keep you and your wife in my thoughts and prayers. You're pretty fucking stubborn (if I remember right) so I don't see something like cancer beating you!

Trey to Dani D, Jan 30, 2006

Hah, someone who remembers me from junior high and high school. Trust me, "pretty fucking stubborn" is pretty much an understatement from those days.

Thanks for the note, Dani, it's good to hear from you. I hope all is well with you. And it won't be cancer that gets me, it'll be something way more interesting: bad fruit in a third world country, getting run over by a drunk Irishman in County Derry, getting shot by the irate mother of one of my inmates, that kind of thing.

Part 15
January 30, 2006 – 2:06 pm

Tom Piccirilli sent me a note recently (and if you want to know why I want to be Tom when I grow up, check out damn near anything he's written) and he made a great point.

Basically, quit whining.

Okay, that's only the most superficial way to have read his email, but that's how it hit me. I sent him a note bitching — again — about the side effects of the shots and he wrote back, saying he understood the three times a week shots were tough, but weren't they better than the daily treatments?

In other words, as long as the side effects aren't as bad as December, then my situation is getting better.

In still other words, quit whining.

He's most definitely right. I realized I was getting into a complaint funk. Don't get me wrong, I'm still going to complain — it's what I do best — but overall, I'm in a better position than I was in December.

I knew that, obviously, but sometimes I guess I'll need a little reminding.

Why? Because I'm so tired of being tired. Because all I really want is to be normal again. Don't want to have to worry about eating at the right time (an hour before a treatment so I can take the medicine), or should I drive or not, do I need to call in sick, can I remember my wife's name, etc.

(And yeah, I realize my bitching is fairly well petty compared to people in stage 4 lung cancer or with heart failure or Alzheimer's, but there it is.)

I just want to go back to the end of November before it started. Except not really then because I was healing from lymph node surgery then. Maybe September, then. Except not really then because that's when the lymph node was swollen to its largest and most painful.

I guess I want to go back to when I was ten and didn't have a single damn care in the world except getting to the skating rink and hoping Robby's mom (a tall hot blond who owned the rink) was there in those incredibly tight Jordache jeans she used to wear.

Welcome to ten years old; "I ain't sure what I'd do with it, but it sure looks great in those jeans!"

What I'm saying is over all, compared to others with cancer, I'm doing pretty well, even if I have to rant sometimes.

Actually, a dispatcher at the Sheriff's Office put it more succinctly: shut up about it or die already.

She laughed so I'm pretty sure she was joking.

I don't know…maybe not…they're a pretty tough crowd.

Comments

Scanner Darkly, Jan 30, 2006

Heh. Yeah. Does indeed sound like a tough crowd.

IMHO — people bitch a lot more about things when they are only annoying or frustrating, rather than terrible. Daily treatments is the constant reminder that you're fighting against death. Treatments three times a week is still big, but it has more of that irritation thing.

But then again, I've always thought Lily Tomlin was right when she said "Sometimes I wonder if humanity developed language out of a deep inner need to complain."

Tom Piccirilli, Jan 31, 2006

Sorry you interpreted my email as "quit whining". I certainly never meant for anything I sent to sound like a) you were or b) that you should stop if you were. Merely that I was glad that things seemed to be getting better for you as time went on. Considering I'm a grade-a bitcher, and bitch about everything in my life whether its worth it or not, I wouldn't ever tell somebody else they didn't have the right to vent. Especially when they were feeling upset about some pretty damn scary things. But I also know how easy it is to fall into depression and despair, so it's good to try to see the bigger picture if you can. Sometimes we all need reminding of that to help us stay in a positive mindset, which can only help.

Pic

Trey to Tom, Jan 31, 2006

Tom, absolutely no apologies needed. I realize you didn't write quit whining, but that my emotional baggage let me read it.

It was exactly what I needed to read, exactly what I needed to hear. You were dead right: things are getting better, they are looking up. It is exactly what I said in the later post about Wendy Wasserstein: my situation is minor compared to her daughter's.

That was the only point I was trying to make. The problem was, I tried to use a bit of humor and we all know ain't no way I oughta be writing no funny stuff 'cause it just ain't funny.

Debbie B, Feb 1, 2006

I printed out your whole journal and read it last night. And I disagree with you…you are funny. I can't believe we're the same age. WTF is wrong with you? Cancer? A heart attack? It was probably due to all the Taco Villa you ingested while growing up in Midland. No, that can't be it…I ate Taco Villa. I know what it is…your body is rejecting you for leaving the great State of Texas. Yeah, that's the ticket.

In any case. I don't know if you pray. I don't know if you even believe. But I do, so I will pray for you.

Take care my friend.

Tina F, Feb 15, 2006

I have to agree with Debbie, you ARE funny! You and your wife are in my prayers. She's one helluva lady to put up with you….LOL

Keep writing! I love knowing someone famous!

Part 16: Hydration, anyone?
February 8, 2006 – 3:51 pm

So here's what happened:

I got a shot about 10:30 yesterday morning, then headed to work. Not overly worried because my dizzy/lightheadedness doesn't usually happen until about four hours after my shot, and it's usually pretty mild.

Hah. Not this time.

At 11:15, we got the inmates out for lunch. I was standing in a room full of prisoners and more than a couple of them looked at me as though my face were sliding off my skull.

Then I felt a little dizzy. I sat down next to an inmate I didn't know and that seemed to freak him out a little (didn't like a guard sitting right next to him while he was eating, I guess). I got dizzier and dizzier until I finally banged on the main door to get out of the lunch room and into the empty booking room. I sat in a chair and then woke up a few minutes later with something like 18 or 20…or maybe 30 or 35…deputies standing around staring down at me.

And they were all real tall. Which told me I was on the floor.

Almost immediately, their jokes started. And yeah, they were all at my expense. I wouldn't have expected anything else.

I don't remember much else until I woke up in the ambulance. I remember bits and pieces of conversation and I think I remember sitting on the floor under a blanket maybe crying a little (Not my usual, screeching like a third grade girl kind of crying, but something a bit more dignified…snot running outta my nose kind of thing.)

LuAnn was already there, having come to the jail to bring me some meds and somehow managed to time her visit just right.

In the ER, I got poked and prodded and they stole a pile of blood, and didn't want me to go to sleep just yet (I was really tired). The only good moment was when four or five nurses were around me, doing their schtick, and one of them said, "I bet you haven't ever had this many women touching you at once, huh?"

What I should have said was what Ed Gorman said to me when I told him this story, "Well, not with their clothes on," but I was pretty well too foggy to say anything coherent and Ed didn't toss me the line until the next day.

Diagnosis? Not enough fluids. Not enough food. Not enough sleep.

Food and fluids yeah yeah, I've been hearing it for two months. But sleep?

The last couple of weeks, the winter dryness and the Interferon have dehydrated me so badly that my skin crackles when I walk. Everything itches and it doesn't matter how much lotion I use. I'm lucky to get three hours sleep right now.

The ER doc told me to talk to my oncologist and get a Benedryl prescription, then I should be good to go.

All in all, a very odd day. But the best part, aside from the fantasy of five nude nurses, was the doctor's note I got: "Dear Sheriff, please excuse Deputy Barker from work for two days."

If I just keep changing the date on that note, I might be able to use it whenever I want to stay home and think about those nurses.

Comments

John P, Feb 8, 2006

Wait, what's the incentive to stay out of the hospital now?

(Humor aside, though, still worried aboutcha, bud.)

Lori M, Feb 9, 2006

No matter how many drugs they give you or how many times your body breaks down to get your attention, you will never change! There you were lying in the hospital, barely conscious, and you were thinking about the nurses. I don't know how LuAnn puts up with you. Oh well, I'm glad you are still the same old Trey I remember. Take care of yourself, I want my sons to meet you someday.

My love,

Lori M (Chris' wife, your long lost Texas friends)

Mom, Feb 9, 2006

You sure are getting friendly with all the floors in town, son. Maybe you should take up posing for Febreeze ads.

Trey to Mom, Feb 11, 2006

There it is folks. My mom. If that whole mom thing doesn't work out for you, you can get a gig in comedy. Febreeze. Hah.

Grandmother Smith, Feb 9, 2006

Trey, I haven't sent any comments previously because I can't think of anything interesting or amusing to say. Just "I care about you" and "I'm praying for you". I hope when you are well again you will be able to make a trip back this way and maybe we can find something weird and grabbing for you to write about here in my town.

Trey to Grandmother Smith, Feb 11, 2006

Your emails have been wonderful, Grandma. I appreciate the sentiments but you might want to draw back on that offer of digging up odd stuff to write about. I'm high maintenance when I'm on a writing mission. I might annoy the crap out of you.

Trey to Lori, Feb 11, 2006

Wow, there's a blast from the past. Lovely Lori and her equally good looking hubby Chris. Thanks so much for dropping by and dropping a line, I've missed you guys. I hope all is well with all of you. Email me and help me catch up.

And yeah, you didn't really think I'd think about anything other than the women, did you? Maybe the bills and maybe — No, the women.

Ellen D, Feb 12, 2006

Trey,

Just catching up on reading friends' live journals after being away (in Prague) for almost a week. Sorry to hear about this extra little scare.

Hang on in there. I'm thinking of you.

Part 17: Better Living Through Pharmaceuticals
February 11, 2006 – 12:30 am

Ah, drugs...I love 'em.

Got a prescription for some anti-itch thing yesterday. Took a pill before bed and slept damn near all the way through the night. No itching, no scratching, no zombie-like being awake all night long. Best night of sleep I've had since the shots started in January.

Whoooo-whooooo! I love it.

Hydrohoopteeoxydoodle or some shit. I don't know what it is, I just like taking it. I guess I should find out what I'm destroying the temple of my body with. On the other hand, I'm sleeping so who the shit cares?

Drawback is that the pills will make me sleepy. Nurse told me that and I thought, of course it will, everything about this cancer crap makes me sleepy or fatigued.

But to be honest, in this one case, inducing sleep is good.

***

Once the docs – and five nude nurses — were finished with me at the ER the other day, I turned over, curled into a fetal position, and went right the hell to sleep. I woke up at one point and LuAnn was standing there.

Then I went back to sleep. Woke up later and C–, Ben Atkinson's wife (Ben who likes to call me retard) was standing there. Went back to sleep. Woke up later and Ben was standing there, calling me retard.

Ben later wondered if I thought I had died and everyone was taking turns at the viewing.

Yeah, thanks for that, Benny Bo-Fenny. Really appreciate the support.

Can't yell at him too badly, though, he has gotten me home a number of times and bought lunch a whole lotta times.

All in all, I'd like to keep him outta my house. But in such a way that he'll continue to buy lunch.

Comments

Scanner Darkly, Feb 11, 2006
....five nude nurses?

Ellen D, Feb 12, 2006
You missed the post from the 9th!

Scanner Darkly, Feb 12, 2006
Ooohhhhhh. I did! That's what I get for avoiding livejournal for a week.

Part 18: The Treatment Room
February 17, 2006 – 3:33 pm

During December, I got daily Interferon treatments. Most days, it was done in an ambulatory services room at Perry Memorial Hospital. But every Thursday, I went to my oncologist's clinic.

Lots of exam rooms, a nice lobby, a nice little lab for mixing meds, a great little reception room with pleasant nurses who kept the office humming.

But there was another room, at the far end of the hallway, tucked away literally at the end of the road in that suite of offices, that the nurses called the treatment room.

The first thing I noticed was the medical equipment. It wasn't like the hospital rooms where you expect to see thousands of dollars of medical-industrial gear. This stuff, IV stands, miles and miles of medical tubing, hundreds of alcohol swabs and syringes, Band-Aids, butterfly closures, bags of IV solution, stood out like a cluster of cancer cells on a PET scan. And it all stood out because the treatment room was so obviously — so strenuously — not a hospital room.

The walls were painted bright white, trimmed in yellow wallpaper borders that were covered in bouncy little vines and flower petals. On the walls were prints of summer scenes and every single print had something to do with water. The beach scenes had cabanas and sun umbrellas and sand castles, all were drenched with golden sunlight or clear blue skies.

The harbor scenes were filled with small pleasure craft, the kind of thing that two people — a couple, maybe — could easily take out for a day on the water, or take to their favorite hidden beach and pass the day away.

The style of the prints was that overly precious, cloying — and annoying — country style that just makes me want to vomit. You know, on wooden bits of furniture it includes cut-out hearts, colors always pleasant without having any edge. It's the style that has lots of cats and jars of preserves and funny sayings posted above the outhouse door. Entirely too drenched in sweetness for me.

It all freaked me out; the blast of yellows and light blues, of pastel pinks and greens, of just so much goddamned sunshine. It was like my oncologist was trying to enforce happiness on me; as though if he pushed pleasant little outdoor scenes hard enough, I'd forget I was getting chemo for stage 3 cancer.

But the people made me remember.

There were no people in any of the prints.

Not a single person in any of the boats or cabanas, or lounging in the sand, or looking for starfish.

No people. As though everyone had died.

But there were people in the treatment room. It was usually rife with people, in fact. Mostly women, mostly old, and all showing pictures of their grandkids, of the last vacations they took, of the new carpet or interior paint job in their house.

They were the people who should have been in the pictures. At least, they were trying to be those people. They were all about sunshine and clear sky, all about laughter and going on a picnic and opening presents at Christmas time and watching their grandkids graduate from high school.

They were never pissed off, never sad, never resigned.

And of course, they were always pissed off and sad and resigned. But those women — none of whom I could ever bring myself to talk to — were living versions of those pictures.

The paintings had all been done specifically in bright, happy colors and the women were the same. They painted themselves in the same bright, happy colors to mask everything going on inside them. To mask the sickness and the bleeding and the two or four or seven bags of chemo hanging at their sides, to mask the two or three or four hours spent every day with chemo bubbling through their systems.

But all of it — the paintings and the wallpaper border and the women, especially the women — were too much. It was all trying too hard, and that only served to highlight the cruelty of both the room and the situation.

I hate that room.

I don't ever want to go back.

Comments

Grandmother Smith, Feb 19, 2006

Trey, if ever I had any doubts about whether you could write, they are moot now. This entry in your journal seemed to wring my heartstrings and by the time I had finished reading it, I was in tears and for a long time afterwards.

Part 19: By Thine Own Hand
March 4, 2006 – 1:47 pm

It's always so much better when you use your own hand and you're alone.

Hehehehe…that boy is so nasty.

Today was the first day of giving myself the shots. I've been looking forward to doing that for a while now, but it took a few weeks to get all the paperwork through.

Last Thursday, I get a delivery and suddenly my refrigerator is full of drugs and syringes. This morning I went to the hospital, they taught me how to give the shots and off I went.

This will be much better. I'll give the shot before I go to sleep so the lightheadedness and weakness and all the rest will happen while I'm sleeping. Hopefully, this will make me more functional during the day.

But one thing I hadn't thought about is disposal of the syringes. Technically, once they're used, they're medical waste. Can't just toss them in the garbage. So I got an empty gallon milk jug and I'll throw them in there, then take them to the hospital or somewhere for disposal.

Giving the shot wasn't so tough, not as tough as I thought it would. Generally, I'm a wuss; hate pain. The thought of giving myself the pain, whether or not I could stab myself, had left me with some trepidation. But I told myself to quit whining and just get it done. I swabbed myself down with alcohol wipes, pinched up some fat, and jammed the needle in. A pinch of pain and a little sting as the Interferon went in, but other than that, it was no problem at all.

So now I could be a certified heroin junkie.

The shots will go until December, then I'll be finished with everything assuming the cancer doesn't come back this year…and if it does come back, I'm getting my money back 'cause obviously the treatments didn't work.

***

My dreams are still strange. Three or four dreams a night that are absolutely non-sequiturs, have no context to anything going on in my life right now. For instance, the only one from last night that I can remember was me standing in my shower, unable to stand up because those little rubber mats stuck to the bottom of the shower were gone. I kept slipping and falling.
WTF?
I should have been keeping a journal of just the nightly odd dreams 'cause they're all kinds of strange.

***

The Treatment Room. One of the nurses and I were talking about it the other day. I told her how depressing I thought the room was. She told me that until a couple of years ago, there had been no pictures at all. But a prominent Princeton resident (in other words, someone with a healthy ego and bank account to match) had complained and demanded some art work.
One of the first pictures — the beginning of the beach theme, I guess — had two extremely obese women wearing bikinis. That picture evidently offended everyone so they got rid of it and got the pictures that are there now.
I'd just as soon have had the fat chicks picture. At least that would have been funny…like the poster that came with Queen's "Bicycle Race," hundreds of big women on bikes.
Except if I remember correctly, the Queen poster was naked chicks.

***

On the good news front, the doctor told me I didn't have to come back any time soon. He'd been seeing me every two or three weeks. At my last appointment, he said everything looked "extremely good." He said I don't have to go see him for two months.

As far as I'm concerned, that's huge. Maybe I'll get out of this alive after all.

***

That's about it for now. In fact, unless something interesting happens — passing out while driving, passing out while fighting a drunk in the jail, finding a lump the size of Montana on the backside of my head — there won't be anymore Chronicles on anything approaching a regular basis.

Except maybe I'll start keeping a listing of the odd dreams. Who knows, maybe now I'll dream about fat chicks in bikinis.

Whooo-hooo!

Comments

Claudimp on Mar 4, 2006

Unsolicited & gratuitous advice: Might be able to get a sharps container from the drug store — they need to keep them for diabetics, usually. Failing that, think thick plastic — e.g., an orange juice bottle that it'd take a 19-year-old in Doc Martens to even half-crush. The ideal is something where, if the cap comes off inside the bottle and the point pings against the plastic, the plastic shouldn't even notice

All the best with the interferon — it's a tough one, I did it, though I don't know your dosage — but you do get through. May all your cancer cells die in unspeakable agony. (I mentioned to the nice lady at the clinic that I visualized my viruses writhing in unspeakable torment, as though I'd just poured SuperLye all over them. She gave me the oddest look. Don't think this is what they'd had in mind by encouraging me to Think Positive.)

Ellen D, Mar 6, 2006

So glad you're here again. You hadn't blogged in so long I was beginning to worry.

Trey to Claudimp, Mar 7, 2006

Thanks for the advice. Luckily, at my jail, we have a handful of sharps containers. So I just stole one from there and everything's cool. I'm sorry, did I say stole? From a jail? I meant borrow…on a more or less…permanent…basis.

Thanks, too, for your kind words about unspeakable agony! It's good to have the support of friends who mention me and unspeakable agony in the same breath!

Trey to Ellen D, Mar 7, 2006

I think part of it, honestly, is that I've been feeling pretty good the last couple of weeks. So when I have a little time to myself, rather than sitting at the computer, I've been outside doing the things I couldn't do for twelve weeks.

It is a problem in terms of my writing, though. Now that I have some energy to sit down and work(and fiction writing takes much more out of me that non-fiction…making it all up versus simply reporting), all I want to do is sit on the front porch, sun on my face, Corona in hand, and read other people's fiction.

Part 20
Tuesday, March 14th, 2006

I'm writing right now through the haze…or what I think of as The Haze.

I had a shot a little bit ago and I'm a little lightheaded. So if I pass out while writing this, someone call 911.

Okay, okay, not funny.

The news is good on the chemo front. I've begun taking the shots myself at home, usually a couple hours before I hit the sack and it's been fabulous. I don't suffer through as many of the side effects — lightheadedness or dehydration or whatever. And when I do have them, they aren't as bad.

In fact, I've had enough energy to get back to exercising, which, in turn, gives me more energy. And with more energy, I've finally gotten back to writing some fiction. Yeah yeah yeah, I can hear the moans of 'delight' from all my fans out there.

Another big plus? The itching isn't as bad.

So all in all, things are going well right now. Finally. I hate having to stab myself twice for each treatment, but I'll do it if it means avoiding the other problems.

But my dreams are still strange. Hehehe…that's not really a problem. Call it more of an interesting exercise in gonzo film making or experimental theater.

Usually, for the first hour or so after I wake up, I'm a little off-balance. Maybe it's because during the worst of the side effects, I'm asleep and not eating or taking fluids. It's not bad, just a little disconcerting. I haven't fallen or stumbled down the stairs or anything.

Overall, I still get tired. In fact, at the jail last week I worked about 70 hours and then spent most of yesterday sick.

Are those two things related? I've no idea but I suspect so. Today I feel pretty good.

Except now I'm in The Haze. I had to take today's shot early because it looks like I'll have to go in tonight to cover a shift.

As I think about it, this seems like an especially boring dispatch from the cancer world. That's both good and bad. Good because it means I'm doing much better. Bad because it means I have nothing interesting to write about as concerns the Chronicles. No sitting in the road, no passing out in the jail, no time spent in the treatment room.

Wow, it seems I might actually survive all this after all.

That's good, I guess, though I suspect most of my family wouldn't have been particularly bummed out. I mean, I've got pretty good life insurance coverage.

Part 21
Sunday. March 19th, 2006

My wife is a very sensual woman. Her touch. Her hair. Her incredible eyes. And those touching words: "You're looking pretty scrawny."

Ah…thanks, honey…I feel so much more sexy now.

The weight continues to melt away. Last time I was weighed I was down about 25 pounds. It's closer to 30 or 35 now and that's fine, except I have lost — and continue to lose — muscle mass.

That scares me a bit on any number of levels, not the least of which is that sometimes I have to fight with drunks and idiots in my job. Much harder to prevail in a fight if I can't lift my fist. I guess if the fight comes my way, I'll have to hand out IOUs: "Come see me in two months for an ass-kicking."

And obviously the exercising doesn't go anywhere near as quickly as I would like. I want to work out a couple three or four times and be back where I was. Ain't happening. Hell, it took months to lose the muscle, it'll take just as long to get it back.

Part of the problem is the constant fatigue. The chemo, as I've said before, keeps me tired. I keep thinking it'll get better, maybe as I get used to the dosage or whatever. But I've been on this dosage now for weeks and the fatigue hasn't changed.

And I've noticed that if I'm already tired or sick when I take a shot, the side effects hit me much harder.

Last week, for instance. It was a tough week at the jail; lots of jailers sick, lots out injured. There were tons of hours that had to be filled and I ended up working better than 70 hours.

I was exhausted and Thursday and Saturday's shot left me lightheaded, dizzy, and throwing up. Those shots pounded me pretty badly and I can only believe it was because of being so tired.

When I get a good amount of rest, the shots aren't too bad. It's like I've come to a place where I can tolerate them as long as I don't think I'm healthy, as long as I don't think I can do what I used to.

As long as I remember I'm fighting cancer.

Perhaps that level of fatigue, regardless of how I eat or how much I sleep, is where I'll be for the next nine months, until I'm quit of this shit.

There is something else interesting I've noticed, too: growing aggression.

In my jail, I'm the talker. I'm the one trying to solve problems without resorting to violence. I've got so much patience even drug counselors would roll their eyes.

But not lately. Lately, I'm ready to throw-down at the slightest reason.

Inmates get mouthy with me on a regular basis, it's a basic part of the job. Before I started chemo, I'd shrug it off, laugh it off, toss an insult back at them, whatever.

Rarely did anything they said rise to the level of getting physical or even getting physically intimidating.

But now it's hard to keep myself in check. I found myself yelling at a drunk, ready to go around with him when he said he knew where I lived and would come find me.

Of course he didn't know where I lived and even if he had, he didn't remember the threat two minutes after making it. He was a drunk idiot who was just babbling, yet I wanted to kill him.

Am I more aggressive because of the medicine? Or because I'm so tired all the time?

Probably a little of both.

But I do know I'm irritated sometimes because people are idiots. A few nights ago, a co-worker said I — and my medical problem — was the reason the county's self insurance would go bankrupt. "Big claims like yours," she said. "They won't have the money to pay them."

You know, when I'm on my way back from the bathroom where I've spent ten minutes vomiting, when I'm working my fifth or sixth straight 12 hour shift, when I'm unsure about can I navigate the stairs, maybe telling me I'm going to break the county isn't the way to go.

Luckily, I have LuAnn. When I have a bad day, I can stand in front of her, strip, and get those sultry words: "You're looking pretty scrawny."

I'm sure that'll pick me right up.

Part 22: A Long-Lost Death
March 23, 2006 – 10:56 am

It was just a cold.

Except it wasn't just a cold and now his funeral is Saturday.

I never really knew my biological father. I knew the stories about him and the fears of him, but not the man himself. He was gone before I was barely out of diapers, disappeared in the west Texas wind.

Occasionally, the wind would blow some hint of him back toward me. There were stories from my parents' mutual friends that even as I hit eight, nine, ten years old, he was still flashing a picture of an 18-month old me like it was a new picture.

Sometimes he'd call. Left one message when I was in high school that I should call him. Except the number turned out to be a dry cleaner's in Little Havana.

A couple years before that, he called a number of times in just a few weeks. Scared my mother so badly (she thought he was coming for me) that she borrowed a gun from a police officer friend of hers. This woman, who is absolutely, vehemently anti-gun, borrowed a revolver and was fully prepared to lay that hammer down over and over until it clicked on an empty chamber.

That was the first time I realized how scary Clint was. That was the first moment I understood the beatings and the lies, the tyranny.

And in the face of all that, all I wanted to do was meet him. Failing that, I just wanted to know him. I wanted to understand everything about this man who had taken my incredibly strong mother and turned her into a quivering mass of dead scared.

So frightened of him, in fact, that there was a standing order at the Midland Independent School District. No one, Mom ordered, was to ever take me out of class. She and she alone would take me out of class if needed. No one, she further ordered, was to take me out of class based on a phone call or a note.

She was terrified Clint might snatch her up, put a gun to her head, and demand she call the school for his son.

I had no idea of the school order until a few weeks ago. I'm working on another project and as Mom and I talked about that, the school order came up.

In the late '90's, I became interested in my connection to the Kelleys. I began to do research into Clint's family, thinking him to be long dead. Eventually, I discovered he was very much alive, living in Charleston, South Carolina.

That first phone call was the most torturous phone call I've ever made. At that point, it had been 30 years for us. We talked for a couple hours and what drives me a little nuts, even six years later, is that the first phone call was exactly like all the stories, all the anecdotes. He was full of himself, constantly telling me what a great man he was, how smart he was, how on top of the world.

Every fucking word outta his mouth was a lie; built on some tiny wisp of truth, then embellished until the truth was crushed beneath the weight of the imaginary.

The picture, for instance, of the tiny baby being carried by the Oklahoma City fireman after the bombing of the Murrah Building was taken by one of my cousins.

Bullshit. Yes, my cousin is a photographer. Yes, the last name of the actual photographer was the same. But it wasn't my cousin.

Why the lie? My mother believes it was the only way Clint could live with himself. That he knew his life was crap, that his existence had been a disaster front to back. That he filled the many cracks and crevices of his life with the kind of life he wanted rather than the life he had.

And yeah, he was abused and neglected as a child but at some point, don't you have to take control? At some point, don't you have to take responsibility?

He had wanted to meet me a million times between August, 2000 and March 19, 2006. He constantly sent me emails asking where we could meet, when we could get together. He had friends in Chicago and made a number of trips to the Windy, always asking to see me.

I never went.

In September, 2005, he made reservations in Chicago for Bouchercon, a mystery convention I attended. I told him not to come. I told him I had to do business, had to meet agents and editors and other writers, told him I had to network my newly published first novel and it would be difficult if he and I were exploring each other.

He stayed home and there is a huge part of me that will forever writhe in guilt over that. It was, though I couldn't know it, the last time we'd have a chance to see each other.

The last time because a few weeks later he was diagnosed with cancer.

I don't remember what kind, though he told me. At first I blew it off. He was such a liar, and he told me about his after I told him about mine. It just didn't feel true. It had the ring of so many of our conversations: yeah, you might have done this, son, but I did it first and better. You might have this affliction, but I do, too, and mine is much worse.

Turns out his was worse. As I got healthier, he got sicker. As I learned to cope with chemo, his tongue swelled and burned from radiation.

As I discovered how to live with my cancer, he understood he was going to die from his.

He died after refusing any more radiation. He got a cold and it slipped into his lungs.

His cancer scares the shit outta me. First and foremost, it scares me. He died from this thing I have, although a different form, and what does that mean for me? It's selfish and self-involved but that's where my head is right now.

I find I'm also covered in guilt, like dirt blown against me by that west Texas wind into which he disappeared. I should feel worse about his death. I should feel guilty about always putting him off, about refusing to meet him until I could arrange it on my terms rather than his.

But I don't. I'm sorry I put him off in Chicago but beyond that, there doesn't seem to be much guilt or sadness.

Just fear. He had a heart attack. I had a heart attack. He died from cancer. I have cancer with something like a 60 percent chance it'll come back.

I asked him once why he left the dry cleaner's number in Miami. He had no idea, didn't even remember calling me. And as far as I know, he long ago lost the picture of me at 18-months.

Comments

Scanner Darkly, Mar 23, 2006
>That's a hell of a post, there.

Dani D, Mar 23, 2006
>You know, Trey, I met my birthmom. It's not all its cracked up to be. I actually went to live with her when I was 21. I had been on my own since the last few months of our senior year. So it was a shock to the old system. She passed away this summer. When I first met her I was really excited. When I got to know her I was really sad. Man she was NUTS.

I don't know if I am better off from knowing her or not. But I realized after many years of knowing her I would of been totally screwed up being raised by a psycho like her. (Not that I'm not a little screwed up from living with my foster parents, I won't mention any last names). But she was a total nutbag. And lied, man she lied all the time. She would lie about anything. She would even lie about the weather. It was weird.

She was so ridden with guilt about abandoning my brother and I. She could not deal with life unless she was high. She could not look me in the eye and towards the end she was so ridden with guilt every time I talked to her she would cry and apologize. In the 60's and 70's she was addicted to drugs. In the 80 she switched to pharmaceutical drugs. When she died she took the answers to all the questions I had for her. She never answered any of them, at least coherently. No matter how many times I asked her for answers I never got any. Her life was so sad to me and her death was even sadder. She overdosed on pain Vicodin and soma. Maybe on purpose maybe not.

When I went to her funeral everyone wanted me to get up and speak about my mother. I didn't though. You know they were expecting something nice to be said and I really had nothing nice to say. What do you say? Well folks she was a lyin', child leavin' bitch. But she was my mother and I loved her sort of. But I didn't like her very much. Just did not seem appropriate.

I think you have a stronger will to live then maybe your dad did. You have more to fight for and more to live for.

Diorling, Mar 23, 2006

Some people need to die, in order for us to feel better about them. In death, there is no expectation; all is done, all is quiet except for talking memories…and with time, even those get a bit blurred. A lot of shitty people with an ounce of remorse lie…they'd rather you believe the lie than the shittyness. If you take a written tally about all the things he lied about and only write down the lie, you'll see the man he wished he could appear to be for you. A slight positive intention amidst a landful of dung, and a sad one…but worth the vision just the same. At the end, just remember, death is never a mistake. Now you can feel a certain peace over never having to wince when the phone rings, and he asks to see you again.

Sean D, Mar 24, 2006
>Fine words, my friend.

Weston O, Mar 27, 2006
>So much of what you said resonates with what I've had to come to terms with. I want to get personal. shoot me an email.

Trey to Sean D, Mar 29, 2006
>I 'magine ol' SD is getting to where he hates calling me. He calls, I tell him I have cancer. He calls, I tell him my publisher dropped me. He calls, I tell him my sperm-donor died.
>Pretty soon, he's going to figure out to quit calling me.

Trey to Weston O, Mar 29, 2006
>Get personal? Not without dinner and desert and maybe some dancing. I may be cheap but I'm not easy.

Weston O, Mar 29, 2006
>Oh come on. What about the night at the Masquerade Jello Twister Party in Boulder. I was the one in the Howdy Doody Costume that tasted like grape nehi.

Trey, Mar 30, 2006
>Yeah, you guys who read this and think it's made up need to go to a few more writers' conventions. Hehehehe....

Marie from Boston, Dec 5, 2006
>Hi Trey,
>You've never actually met me, but I'm almost 100% positive Clint told you all about me – I'm Marie from Boston, and guess what...I do exist! I stumbled across your journal – imagine that! Glad to hear your cancer is in remission – but I also wanted to respond to your post regarding Clint's death. You really only knew the side of Clint that you were told about. Let me tell you the side of Clint that I knew. This man was kind, caring, yes he had a past ...but, everyone deserves a chance to

change and to be forgiven. I am truly blessed (and no I'm not a bible thumper) but I do know that I was blessed to have had the opportunity to know Clint. I cannot even begin to list how special a friend he was to me — A friend who would stay on the phone all night to ease my broken heart when the love of my life was gone, his only motive friendship and concern — he wouldn't say a word other than, "Honey I'm here if you need to talk, I'll stay with you until I hear you snoring." A friend who though nothing of plunking down $1,000 for a Chihuahua puppy to fill the hole in my heart (Perhaps you were lucky enough to hear the antics of Spike the super Chihuahua aka "Leaky") I've traveled to so many places that I might never have had the opportunity to see…if it weren't for Clint. South Carolina, New York City, and heck I even got to see my own City, Boston, thru Clint's eyes…….who knew how great it was! Anyhow, perhaps you resent this post – maybe you're angry or maybe your amused…I'm not a mind reader…so I really don't know. But I will tell you this; Clint really taught me the meaning of true friendship. Oh, and one more thing…if he ever shared the stories about being run over by pink sneakers, or me overflowing the jacuzzi tub in NYC and blaming it on Emmie, or the fact that I absolutely HATE grits, boiled peanuts and the wiggly worm ride — they are all true.

    The best to you and yours.

Trey to Marie from Boston, Dec 10, 2006
    Marie,
    Yes, I've heard quite a bit about you, actually.
    I have to say, I'm shocked you stumbled across the journal, seems so random and odd. But you saw it so that's good.
    Thanks for your kind words about my cancer, I appreciate them.
    < < You really only knew the side of Clint that you were told about. >>

What I was told and what I learned from talking to him a few times a month for five and a half years. As I said in the piece, I believe Clint's reality was somewhere between what Mama told me and what he told me. He was neither as bad nor as good as either of them would have me believe.

I'm glad he was able to become such a close friend for you; that he was able to help you when the clouds were darkest. And $1,000 for a Chihuahua? That's pretty impressive. Unfortunately, he and I were never able to get to that point, for a variety of reasons.

And no, I don't resent the post, nor am I amused by it. It simply is. It's another reminder that people are more complex and multifaceted than we can imagine.

Part 23: Of Coffins and Insurance Companies
April 1, 2006 – 4:34 pm

(this is pretty close to the actual phone call Friday)

Riiiiiinnnnnng!

"Mmmpphhhhh...."

Riiiiiiinnnnnnnngggggggg!!

"Whaaaa? Mmmpphhhhh...."

Rrriiiiiiinnnnnnnnnnngggggggg!!!!!!!!

"What? Yeah? This is Trey."

"I'm looking for Trey Barker."

"Yeah, this is me."

"Trey, I want to talk to you about coffins. I'm selling them. Scratch and dent coffins. Real cheap."

"What? Sorry, I'm a little foggy, I was asleep. Been sick today."

"Sorry to wake you."

"Less you than someone calling about coffins."

"Scratch and dent. Pretty cheap."

"Sean, is that you?"

"Who?"

"Uh...nothing. Why are you calling me?"

"I've got coffins, real nice coffins."

"Nice? Like Pimp My Coffin?"

"No, no, scratch and dent. I've been calling but no one answers their phone."

"They who?"

"On the list. They wouldn't answer so I called you."

"To sell me a scratch and dent coffin."

"Not unless you need one."

"Uh...don't think so but maybe check back in a few days?"

"Tell me about HauntCon."

"Handicam?"

"HauntCon."

"What in the fuck are you talking about?"

"I've got a few scratch and dent coffins, I thought I might go to the convention, see if I can sell them."

"Why did you call me?"

"World Horror Convention…in San Francisco. Thought you might have an idea about dealer spaces."

"For scratch and dent coffins."

"Yeah, and at Hauntcon, too."

"I've never heard of Hauntcon."

"But you know the World Horror Convention, right?"

"My name's on the Board's website."

"Right, I called from that website. No one else would answer."

"Didn't want to talk about coffins no doubt."

"Right."

"Come on, who is this, really?"

"Uh…maybe I have the wrong number?"

"Maybe. Tell you what, you should call Alan B–, owns Borderlands bookstore in San Francisco. He's the big wheel with World Horror this year. I'm not going — health problems — but he can help you out."

"You're not going?"

"No."

"Health problems?"

"Yeah."

"So, you need a coffin?"

***

I've mentioned before that my insurance company has done pretty well by me since all this started. With the exception of taking too long to decide I could do the shots at home, they've been pretty good.

I hate to say this, because I'm as anti-insurance premium and company as the next Red-Blooded American, but over the last two days, my insurance company has jumped to the top of my Good Guy list.

Originally, I was under the impression my monthly batches of Interferon would come automatically. Surprise surprise, I was wrong. I have to reorder every month, takes a couple of weeks to get in. So I ended up in a situation where the new meds weren't going to be here until Monday while my current batch ran out last Thursday.

Left me with no treatment for today.

So I called the company, explained what was what, asked if I should head to Perry Memorial Hospital (and I'm the only one creeped out by a hospital being named 'Memorial?') to get a treatment.

Without getting too boring, it turned into a nightmare of finances and who actually had the medicine in stock in this little town I've chosen to call home. Too expensive to go to the hospital. No Interferon in stock at my oncologist's local office. None at any of the local pharmacies.

So these two women, Dawn at the insurance company and Lisa at Kirby Henning pharmacy, traded a shitload of phone calls and got me hooked up. Got me the exact meds I needed, the right syringes (remember, I don't like the big ones…they hurt!) and all for FREE!!!

I had already paid for the next month's worth of Interferon and at first, the single treatment was going to cost me $1000 (a week's worth, can't sell it in packs less than that). Then it was going to cost the 20% co-pay. Then just my regular $150 cap. Then Dawn decided that since I'd already paid the $150 for the month, she wasn't going to let me pay anything.

Dawn and Lisa are my current favorite chicks, bending over so far backward their spines probably snapped. All for little 'ol me.

Hell, if the coffin salesman had worked that hard for me, I probably would've bought one.

Comments

T.J. C, Apr 1, 2006

I have noticed that the WHC has a large percentage of people interested in it that will call every single number and email every single address on the site except for the one they need to call or write to. My official recommendation to future conventions will be to make One Point of Contact for all things, and hire a damned message service to direct the calls or something. It's a bit frustrating, but then I remind myself that as stupid as the average person is, by definition half of everyone is even more stupid than that.

At any rate, this made me smile today.

Mom, Apr 2, 2006

You are my favorite eldest son! Thanks for the morning hee-haw.

Part 24
Tuesday, April 11th, 2006

Yesterday, the sun shone.

Not like a metaphoric, I-discovered-something-about-myself kind of crap, but actual sunshine. Temperatures hit nearly 70, nary a cloud in the sky. Nothing but beautiful sunshine everywhere.

I spent most of the day doing what I usually do in the springtime: sitting on the porch, reading. This time it was THE CLOSERS by Michael Connelly. I was out there for probably four hours, sometimes dozing, sometimes reading, constantly relaxing.

What I noticed most was that I felt good.

When all this started, it was the dead of December. Snowy, cold, nasty. Add to that chemo, cancer, weight loss. Part of my depression (and it never got as bad as it could have) was the disease. But part was also winter, clouds and snow, temps down below 20.

But now, while we might still have a snow or two, spring is mostly here and everything seems to have changed.

I don't feel healthy by any means — still tired, still cranky, still weak and fighting random bouts of diarrhea, still with dry skin and minor wounds that will still be minor six months from now — but mentally it's like I've gone to Cancun, found a bevy of bikini-clad beauties and an endless supply of cold Corona.

Can something as simple as the sun, as opening windows closed by winter, actually do that much for my spirit?

Damn straight.

Suddenly, with a single kiss from the sun, the worst of the treatments faded into harsh memory. Stumbling to the hospital day after day, slumping to the street or the floor of Kirby-Henning Pharmacy, is now nothing more than something that might have happened to me long ago. Endless blood tests and the metallic taste in my mouth and the weight loss and all the rest seems like an old photograph, bleached by springtime sun until the painful colors are gone, leaving only the outlines of what it had been.

And yet, even with the sun, there are still problems. Today I decided to mow the lawn. I was hardly strong enough to start the damned machine. The first start of the season is always the hardest, but I stood in my driveway, yanking and yanking and yanking again — for nearly a half hour — until it finally started.

I couldn't get enough arm pull into the yanking. Even with all the exercising I've done over the last weeks, I was very nearly too puny to pull.

Then, when I did get it going, it was all I could do to push the thing around the yard. I found myself winded, aching from thirst, arms tired and legs sore.

And head burned.

My coif started going south in high school, and while I hate people who use the phrase 'cue-ball' or 'chrome-dome,' they're both pretty accurate. At the beginning of every spring, I get at least one major burn.

Peeling skin, impossible to wash what hair I have left because of the pain, impossible to sleep.

When I was mowing, I didn't even think about it. Now I've got a bit of a burn and an immune system beat to pieces. God knows how long it'll take my head to heal.

Guess that makes me a sorehead.

But right now, with the sun out, a light breeze on the air, and a new book to read, I'll take the burn. Because burned or not, things are looking up.

Part 24.5: Dream Oddities
Thursday, April 20th, 2006

Well, the truly bizarre dreams seemed to have slowed down. While that's probably good — might well mean the chemo isn't torching my brain as badly as it was — it's also less interesting.

Here are a couple episodes of late.

LuAnn and I are standing on the edge of a large pit. Call it 100 feet per side, maybe 50 feet deep. All the way around the edge are huge boulders. She and I are climbing around on them, we both slip and fall, and the boulders come down and crush us. Then the dream loops. That tiny little bit of subconscious over and over. I've never seen myself killed so many times. It was a little depressing.

Next up: LuAnn and I are in a small house. Two bad guys are trying to break in. I tell her to call the Sheriff's Office and get some help. Instead, she calls a local businessman and they discuss Kool-Aid. While this is going on, I have a lawnmower blade in my hand, hacking away through the window at the head of one of the bad guys. When a chunk of his skull breaks off, the dream is over.

This stuff is so bizarre.

Part 25: Skinny, Scrawny, Scared
April 20, 2006 – 5:29 pm

And the weight just keeps slipping away.

When this whole thing began, I was a bit better than 200 pounds; call it 205, 207, along in there.

I'm at 168 now.

Twenty pounds, twenty five pounds, maybe even thirty pounds, I could take. Needed to lose a few pounds. But losing close to 40 freaks me out. Even with the exercising — weight training to try and gain some muscle tone back and a bit of walking/jogging — I'm losing weight.

Because I can't eat.

Two things: one, most food tastes okay but has a disgusting after taste. Two, I have absolutely no appetite. The thought of food makes my stomach turn. So consequently, I'm not eating much, leading me to the weight loss that lowers my blood pressure and blood sugar, which makes me feel like crap, which makes me want to eat even less.

Let's hear it for vicious circles.

I tried to mow the lawn recently and almost couldn't get the mower started: not enough arm strength to pull the cord. When I finally did get it started, I had to stop every third or fourth mown row because I was exhausted. At one point, Officer Friendly Ben Atkinson drove by to make sure I wasn't dead in the yard.

Hah, that would have shown him, wouldn't it? No more calling me retard, buddy. Just hook me up with a scratch and dent coffin.

The Interferon treatments are making me crazy, hitting me much harder than they have recently. And for a longer period than in the past. Tuesday, before I'd gotten a treatment, I had to leave work, have someone drive me home. I was light-headed, fuzzy brained, foggy. I couldn't understand much of what the other officers said, couldn't remember the names of some of them.

And that was without a treatment. I got home, took that day's treatment, and was out like a dead man.

Dr. Vukov, my oncologist, believes part of the harshness of the treatments is because I weigh less now. More medicine per pound than when I started. Part of the solution is to give me a week with no treatments, then get me started again with a lower dosage.

I'm all for both of those moves.

Even as I write this, I'm having trouble remembering what I'm writing about or what I even want to say. I'm shaky and fuzzy, light-headed, sweaty (which might be low blood sugar again…damn a good reason to eat up a Milky Way bar), and incredibly nauseous. (if I yack on LuAnn's computer, chances are she'll beat me…normally something I'd dig).

I've been doing chemo for five and a half months now and it's getting harder and harder to see the endgame. Eight more moths and I'll be through. Friends say things like keep my eyes on the prize and remember what this is all for and while I agree with that intellectually, mostly it's bullshit.

All I want to do is go home, crawl into bed, cry like a baby, and hopefully sleep until next December.

What a puss I am.

Comments

Tom P, Apr 22, 2006

You're not a puss at all. You're going through a serious trauma here, both physically and emotionally, and it's bound to take it's toll. As for keeping the weight up, you might try investing in high-protein shakes. Since you're not "eating" they might help to circumvent the nausea. Over the course of a day it's easier to drink 3-4 shakes than it is to have 3-4 meals. Gatorade and high electrolyte drinks and juices might help your system to stablize. When you do eat, eat high-caloric foods. Less chewing/swallowing/tasting but higher caloric intake. Get some meat to stick back on your bones.

I can always send you some pasta fasulli.

Good luck, brother. Let us know if there's anything we can do.

Part 26
April 25, 2006 – 9:31 am

The sun is out, warm on my face though in the back of my head I'm a little worried about sunburn, low immunity and all that. Somewhere, birds are tweeting and dogs are barking. Down the street, at Lincoln Elementary, the kids are out at recess. Across the street, a man is re-roofing his father's house while a Marlboro kind of guy, dressed in Khakis and a tan knit shirt, goes door to door, trying to sell new windows.

Through the living room window, I can see my two mutts. Crashed in the sunlight. Tango's head comes up, her eyes glassy and sleepy. She licks her chops, then falls back to sleep.

I'm sitting on my porch, Dr Pepper at my feet, George Pelecanos' new paperback, DRAMA CITY, in my hand. This is how it's supposed to be. This is my normal spring routine.

Dr. Vukov was onto something when he suggested taking a break from treatment, getting my head back together, letting the needle holes in my gut heal. Yes, I had known I was having a hard time physically; yes, I had understood the depression that was coming over me. But I hadn't realized how far gone I was until I had a few days when it was different.

It's almost hard to describe ("Ain't you a writer, or what?") how perfect yesterday was. I got up early, went and exercised, went and bothered LuAnn at the bookstore…getting hyped up about politics and making really, really funny jokes. I don't think I believe in God, but whoever's in charge couldn't have cranked up a better day for me to have on my first day off from both treatments and work.

Today could be just as cool. I've got lunch planned with a copper friend I've not seen in two years. I've got to work on a novel synopsis for my new agent. It's been raining for hours now — most times I love the rain more than the sun, and most of my chemo tongue is gone.

Yet around the edges, I'm tired. Around the edges, it's impossible to forget what's been going on. Takes more than a couple of days to get the chemo-poison out of my system, I guess.

Yet as brilliant as yesterday was, it was also incredibly illustrative. It made me realize, in a much more brutal way, that I'm not even halfway done with treatment yet, that I've still got six months to go. The break is good, helps me remember what it was like before all this shit and what it'll be like after we're done. But it's tough, too because I know that next Sunday, I'll feel like shit again.

But for the next few days, I'll push that aside, ignore what's coming and concentrate on enjoying the here and now, which, now that I think about it, is exactly opposite where my head is during chemo. Chemo is for the future, making certain I'll be around beyond my next birthday.

It's a good day. It'll be good tomorrow, too. And for a few days after that. Then it'll be bad for a while. Then it'll be over.

Hah! What'll I bitch about then?

Comments

Mom, Apr 25, 2006

Don't worry, you will find something to bitch about. After all, don't you take after your mother?

Feo A, May 2, 2006

I've been hearing all about you. Asking every time your name comes up, how yer doing. My Dad's been double whammied by both Parkinson's and cancer and I don't even know what I can say to him. But I've been putting off telling you that I think about you and your situation and I keep wishing for the best for you.

I'm sorry if this all seems trite. There are a few things I'm not so good at and trying to make folks feel better with problems like yours is one of them.

I've gone through your whole journal here. Funny thing is, I've also had that boulder dream, and when I was recovering from poison too. Being a former world traveler and allergic to bee stings, I've had to go through a fair amount of food and insect/spider poisoning.

Anyway, if nothing else, I just want to add my voice to all of the other folks who come by here and wish you the best as well as a full recovery. It happens. It happens a lot. So why shouldn't it happen to you, right?

Of course, once you ARE better I'm going to make fun of you.

Just so you know.

Trey to Feo A, May 3, 2006

Feo, Feo, Feo.

Thanks so much for your note, I appreciate it. Obviously give your father my best. I can hardly handle the little bit of cancer I have, I can't even imagine what you and he are going through. If there is anything I can do, you let me know.

And don't worry about to trite or not to trite, the main thing is the thought and I'm sure it'd be the same with your father. Don't try to think of anything to say, just talk. Let him hear your voice and whatever you need to say he'll probably hear just in the tone and texture. And if that doesn't work, get his ass drunk.

Very curious about the boulder dream you've had…curiousor and curiousor that it came after being poisoned, too. That's one of those things that if I put it in a story, the editor was make me take it out as unbelievable.

Obviously — OBVIOUSLY — I'd expect, nor want, no less than complete ridicule at your hands…once I'm healthy.

Part 27: Back On The Poison Bus
Wednesday, May 3rd, 2006

Ok, I'm officially back on chemo.

How do I know (aside from giving myself the shots)? Food tastes like shit again and all I wanna do is sleep.

Last week was brilliant. No shots, food tasted decent, soda was good, my sense of humor was back, my sense of political righteousness came back with a vengeance. It was a great week, except a number of deputies were desperate for me to get BACK ON the shots. Something about the jokes not being funny and me having too much energy.

I figured Sunday's shot would be tough on me since I'd been clear for 8 or 9 days. I was right. Hit me hard, hit me fast, but then was gone. Gotta love that lower dosage, right?

Tuesday night's shot didn't hit me at all before I went to sleep. But when I got up this morning, I was kind of light-headed. Not much, just enough to be noticeable, enough to give me pause.

So what'd I do to combat that being light-headed? I went and worked out. Actually did better on my mile and a half walk/jog than I've done since before this all started. Did better on the weights. Now I'm tired, but it's not chemo tired, it's actual tired from doing something.

The side effects of being a passenger on the poison bus have started, but thus far — and it's still early yet in the second half of the chemo run — the lower dosage is good. Still weak, still tired, but not as much as I have been. I think taking a bit less chemo in each treatment will be the best thing that's happened to me in the last few months.

The odd dreams have come back, too. I wake up in the morning and know something goofy's been going on in my brain, but I haven't been able to remember exactly what. Get off chemo, dreams go away, get back on, dreams come back. Post hoc ergo propter hoc. (And no, I don't randomly know Latin, I stole that from 'West Wing.')

Something else has come back, too: my aggression.

Last week it wasn't bad. I didn't want to punch anyone or get in any fights at the jail or whatever. I didn't scream and yell at bad drivers. A good week.

But last night, Princeton Police radioed that they had arrested a drunk. He was big and he was a fighter. Get ready, PPD said.

My stomach dropped. Don't like that fighting thing.

So me and my partner got ready and when the police car pulled up into the Sally Port, we heard him screaming. Mind you, we were inside the jail and he was loud enough that we still heard him.

I went to the car door, opened it, and was absolutely verbally assaulted with all kinds of stupidity. It annoyed me, but not to any great degree, that happens in my job.

I get him out of the car and we're taking him into the jail. That's when he got goofy. Didn't matter he was handcuffed, didn't matter that he was so drunk he could barely walk, he wanted to throw down.

He shoved me a bit, made a few hints toward head-butting me, but nothing really more than that.

Still I'm cool, still I'm not worried about it. Drunks are drunks.

But then he called me a nigger and I lost it. Screaming and yelling at him and, when he came toward me once again, putting him over the squad car's trunk.

I was absolutely infuriated. All I wanted to do was pound him bloody. I have no idea why that word set me off, why I didn't just blow it off like I did everything else he said — faggot, panty-raper, you wanna fuck my ass, I'll kill you and your family with an AK-47, etc — but I didn't.

Luckily, there were enough other offices around for me to back out of the situation without getting completely stupid. My partner and my sergeant handled it, put him to bed and when he sobered up, he was actually apologetic.

And all of that's fine, just another day in the life of a jail guard. But I can't get past my freaking out when he tossed the word nigger out as easily and casually as someone tossing a few quarters into a blind musician's guitar case. Maybe because it was meant to be insulting, maybe because I grew up around that crap and it just makes me nutty. Hell, might even be white man's guilt. Who knows?

All I know for sure is that I was aggressive — and very nearly stupid — and wanted to get more aggressive.

The sad thing is: he could have snapped me like a twig even with the cuffs on.

All of this is just to say: I'm back on chemo. I hate it and all of its side effects but now I'm a few days less than 6 months from finished. I've crossed that line, that point of no return, and I'm completely stoked about that.

A little bit more...then all will be right with the world again...at least my part of the world.

Part 28: Six Months At Most
Thursday, May 4th, 2006

So, Officer Friendly (famed in song and dance as the one who calls me retard when I'm foggy from chemo…and now just randomly 'cause he thinks it's funny) and I went to lunch today.

And he almost killed me in a car accident.

Yeah, that's insulting enough, but when I said don't kill me, he responded with: "Now or in six months, what's the difference?"

Thank you, thank you very much.

I can always look to Sergeant Ben Atkinson for support and I will always appreciate that, even when I'm dead in six months and LuAnn is trying to track down the scratch and dent coffin salesman.

In all seriousness, though, I think the lowered dosage of chemo is going to be extremely good for me. Yeah, I'm still weak. Yeah, I'm still tired. Yeah, I still have lowered blood pressure most days and yes, oh yes, I still get more aggressive than I normally am, but none of it is as bad as it was two weeks ago.

Yeee-hawww! I might survive this bullshit after all.

One thing I have noticed, though, is that this blog posting is less dramatic than it was at the beginning. I went back and read through some of the early posts (which was weirdly sort of navel-gazing-ish) and so often, my writing was so dramatic, edging into melodramatic.

But as the time has rolled past, it seems less so, like the drama of the entire affair is slowly bleeding out. Taking shots every few days isn't anywhere near as dramatic as getting poisoned for an hour a day twenty days running. Talking on the phone to the pharmacy providing the chemo isn't as dramatic as being strapped to a table for surgery or a PET scan. Sitting on the porch and reading Laura Lippman's new novel *No Good Deeds* (a fabulous book, by the by) under a sunny sky isn't as dramatic as watching a roomful of people get bag after bag after bag of chemo.

And for those of you who've read any of my fiction, you know I'm nothing if not overly dramatic.

But maybe part of it, too, is that I'm not as scared as I was. The tests are negative, my oncologist is happy, I see an end to the tunnel I've been in. Whereas weeks ago and months ago all I could see was the cancer and the massive amounts of chemo I had to take to treat it.

I suspect I was much more scared, during the horrible days of late November and all through December, than I admitted. Part of reading the older *Cancer Chronicles* was rediscovering the early dreams, all of which had me in Saturday cliffhanger situations and all of which had me winning in the end. Hmmmmm, I think law enforcement types call that a clue. And I think the clue says I was terrified, beyond even what I told friends and family and probably myself.

Yeah, I'm still a little scared around the edges — after all, even when this is all done it isn't done, I'll have to watch for recurrence my entire life — but it's not debilitating, not paralyzing.

It might be different tomorrow, but today, I believe I'm gonna survive…and if not, then Officer Friendly's comment sounds less like a threat than a prognostication.

Part 29
May 18, 2006 – 12:39 pm

So...I was touching myself today and realized I have a muscle.

Hah, not that one, you disgusting pre-verts.

A few months ago, I started trying to exercise because I realized that I'd become so weak I couldn't even lift meals or supplies at the jail. Nor could I get up the stairs at home without nearly passing out, I was that weak.

Hmmmm, I thought, I have no muscle tone.

So I started very slowly. Walking for a couple of miles, and yeah, it took nearly all day to go that distance. Lifting a few pounds...an embarrassingly few, actually. Recently I added some sit-ups (I figure as long as my gut's gone, I might as well see if there are any ab muscles there...not like a six pack but more like a two and a half pack).

A few days ago, I rubbed the chemo itch on my stomach and realized there was a freakin' muscle there. What the hell? I checked around a little and found things that appear to be muscles in my legs, arms, and my stomach. Wow, like having an actual body. I'm sure the chicks will hit on me right and left. I'll have to beat them off with a stick...or with these incredible muscles I'm packing.

Okay, okay, that's all mostly crap. I'm not muscle-bound, but I'm doing better physically than I have in a little while and that's good. And I'm sure the exercise, particularly the walking/jogging, is helping my immune system and blood counts and all the rest of it.

So that's good news, as is that all my counts look good right now. White blood cells a little lower than where the Doc wants them, but not in scary land yet. Reds and weight (still losing, but not as quickly as before) and lymphs and whatnot all look generally good.

I still have awful days; days when food tastes terrible (and I'm still not eating all that well), days when I'm light-headed, when it's hard to drive or concentrate, nights when I can't sleep because of the side-effects. But overall, the medium days are beginning to outnumber the bad days. I'll let you know when I have a good day.

All of that is tentatively good news. But the best of all possible newses is this: December 2.

The last day. I asked the doctor today and he said we'd stop chemo shots, assuming no massive new outbreak in cancer cells, the week before the anniversary. I started the chemo bullshit Dec. 5, 2005 so Dec. 2, 2006 will be my last day.

Thank the freaking gods. There will be some sort of party on that day. We'll all get together — and that means all the readers in the States, that woman in Australia and the handful in Europe — will come to my house. I'll take the last shot, we'll eat and drink and then you can all laugh at me when I get light-headed (or retarded, depending on how you look at it)!

And no, I haven't yet put a calendar on my wall marking the days off, but I'm sure I will.

I went for a check-up today and Dr. Vukov said he felt like we were just rocking and rolling through all this, that it didn't seem to have been very long since we started, that time was cranking right along.

What the fuck? Try it from this end, cowboy. Time ain't moving so quickly from here.

But maybe it'll move faster now that I have an end date. Or, more likely, it'll slow to a damn crawl as the date gets closer. It'll be like the inmates in my jail. Someone gets sentenced to six months and everything's fine until those last few days. Time damn near grinds to a halt.

So until then, I'll continue touching my muscle and marking the days off the calendar.

Comments

Grandmother Smith, May 22, 2006

Trey, that sounded like pretty good news – I hope you continue to feel better and keep up the exercise. I know it looks like a long road ahead but all things come to an end and I feel this one will have a good end.

Part 30
May 31, 2006 – 2:58 pm

The abuse just keeps on keeping on....

Officer Friendly and I and some intern kid were at a local eatery today and Ben wanted to buy me lunch.

"Why?" I asked.

"Because that way I won't feel guilty about abusing you, retard."

Give him a hand, ladies and gentlemen, my friend, Sergeant Ben Atkinson.

Then, WITHOUT buying me lunch, he goes on ahead with the abuse. Right there! In front of the pizza people! In front of the Princeton PD intern who was looking, I'm sure, for something more professional.

And his grief seemed to give the pizza people the only excuse they needed to abuse me, too!

WTF?

On the other hand, I did get ol' Benny Bo Fenny back a few days ago. He walked into the bookstore and I hugged him.

Then I kissed him.

"What's that for?"

"It's from a woman you've never even met."

I had been on the phone with one of the first girls I ever kissed, Amy K- (she's got a married name now but she'll always be K- to me). I only recently realized she had suffered — and survived — her own bout with cancer. Way back in 1997 and since then, she's been fine and disease free.

It was a great talk. She understood, in the way only catastrophic medical patients can, exactly what had been going through my head for the last six months. She'd heard all the same platitudes, dealt with all the same genuine but uncomfortable moments, had all the same side effects.

It did me a world of good. Not only because I've not seen Amy in eleven years, not only because we'd gone to school together all the way through Midland College and then drifted completely apart, but also because she'd been there. She understood my anger and my mental fatigue and all the rest of it.

She told me she loved what Officer Friendly had done for me, that'd he'd been a close enough friend to insult me to keep me laughing (sometimes at my expense, sometimes at his) when things were rough and ugly. Of course, I don't think she realizes that now he does it 'cause it makes him laugh...my feelings be damned.

She'd had a friend like that, too. Another woman she and I went to school with, Debbie L- (again, there is a married name but to me, Debbie will always be Debbie L-). Ben was my Debbie, the person who tried to keep things as even keeled as possible, however they could.

But Ben wasn't the only one for me. Some of the deputies at the Sheriff's Office, Sean from Omaha, some of the bookstore customers.

(And this has nothing to do with LuAnn or other cancer spouses who offer a completely different, and much more intense support. In LuAnn's case, she didn't have time or energy to insult me because she was so worried about me...you know...not dying.)

I guess the point is, I'm about halfway through this pile of crap — Friday will be six months until the last shot — and I find myself looking backward a little bit. I got through this because of the huge support network I had. There was always someone to help keep me from getting too depressed, or more often in my case, too angry. I appreciate those people and will never be able to repay them for what they've done.

Though I suspect at least some of them will send me some sort of therapy bill 'cause that's how my friends do things.

As for how I'm doing as I take this backward look, most days are good; in fact, there are more good days than bad. At the same time, the bad days are pretty ugly. Last Thursday, a couple hours after my shot, I got incredibly light-headed. Apparently, I almost went head-first down a flight of concrete and steel stairs at the jail. My partner that night snatched me back and another deputy drove me home.

Those days are fewer and further between, which somehow makes them worse when they do happen. If I feel shitty all the time, I don't really notice feeling shitty. But if I feel decent, then I really notice it when I don't. Make sense?

I'm sure that over the next six months, there will be more bad days, but right now, sitting here drinking my Dr Pepper, listening to classic disco, things seem to be okay.

So I tried to tell the pizza people I'd never be back, that I was horrified at my treatment. They laughed — LAUGHED — and said I'd be back because I love their barbequed chicken sandwich.

Damn, they're probably right. Hit me with barbeque, I guess, and you can abuse me all you want.

Comments

Debbie B, Jun 1, 2006

So here I am in Pecos, Texas, in trial, with four law clerk interns that I'm baby-sitting and bored out of my mind as our prison tour has been canceled. I decide to check my e-mail because that's what federal employees do when they're bored. Amy "K" has e-mailed me to read your blog today. You are very kind to mention Amy...she's the best. As for my part in her recovery...she's a bit confused. I didn't do anything. Glad to see you're keeping your sense of humor. By the way, we have something in common...Amy was my first kiss, too. JUST KIDDING!!!!

Anonymous, June 1, 2005
>Every time I see Dr Pepper in one of your post it takes me back to Sonic Drive-In.

>Glad to see you posted I was getting worried. I always worry if it takes you too long to post. Its weird the people who are brought into or back into our lives.

>Take care. Fight the good fight.

Trey to Debbie B, Jun 1, 2006
>Rock and roll! Two chicks kissing! Thanks for the note, Federal Employee, that'll keep me grinning like a pig for days!

>Have fun in trial and thanks for the kind words, I really do appreciate them.

Trey to Anonymous, Jun 1, 2006
>Sonic? Man, does that bring back some memories. Sonic and WhataBurger and Taco Villa, the best fast food joints in all the wide land.

>Now, I'm having a chemo-induced brain fart. I think I know who you are, anonymous poster, but I'm not sure. Give me another clue. Sonic was a good one, as was people brought back into our lives.

>Gimme another.

Trey to Anonymous, Jun 1, 2006
>Damn, now all I want for dinner is Sonic.

Mom, Jun 1, 2006
>You're absolutely right about the shitty days being more noticeable when there are fewer of them. That's the way my hydrops is, kiddo. I think it's the frustration of thinking "hey, I've got this in hand" and then getting hit in the face again.

>Have a Dr Pepper on me, son.

Amy K, Jun 2, 2006

You have to love our Federal Employees! Especially Debbie. She is always modest of her good works. She's the one that is confused. She doesn't think she did anything special because she didn't do anything differently than she ever did.

Deb you promised you wouldn't tell anyone about the kiss!!!

Trey WAS the first boy I ever kissed! Years and miles apart will never change that! You are a special person, you always have been. HALF WAY HOME!!! You are on the downhill slide. I'm having a party all day long in your honor!

Love ya!

Dani, Jun 6, 2006

It was just me Dani. I thought I signed my name. Sorry. I do however like being referred to as anonymous.

Dani, Jun 6, 2006

WE HAVE NO SONICS HERE! THE HUMANITY OF IT ALL!!!

Thank goodness for the new Cherry Vanilla Dr Pepper.

Part 31
June 8, 2006 – 10:30 pm

So the question of the week — since Monday morning in the shower — is "Can I get my money back on the chemo?"

Yeah, I found a lump.

I'm going to the doc's office in a few hours.

Damnit all to hell.

Comments

Scanner Darkly, Jun 8, 2006
...Damn.

Thomas R, Jun 9, 2006
Damn it. I'm sorry.

Lonesome Crow, Jun 9, 2006
Ah, sheesh. Damn it all to hell.

Mom, Jun 9, 2006
Let me know asap, son. I'm keeping my fingers crossed that it's only your meanness bump that you've mistaken for something else.

Morbid Mom, Jun 9, 2006
Oh, no. Hoping for the best!

Aunt M, Jun 9, 2006
Sorry, Trey. We're thinking about you.

Grandmother Smith, Jun 9, 2006

Surely it will be something harmless with all the hopes and prayers your friends and family have had for you. I pray for you twice a day, Trey, and truly believe that you will come out of this OK.

Trey to Mom, Jun 9, 2006

Meanness bump? That's funny. Sadly true, though....

Part 32: A Good Day
June 9, 2006 – 1:33 pm

Ahhhh…the news is good.

"So what's the problem?" the doc asked.

"Well, I've got a lump."

"What do you think it is?"

"Could be cancer."

He nodded. "Yeah, could be."

"Could be a hernia, as much as I've been exercising."

"Yeah, could be."

"Could be a cyst," I said. "I've had them before."

"Yeah, could be."

Okay, Doc, I thought, for as much as I'm paying you, I need something more solid than, "Yeah, could be."

So he copped his regular feel all over my body, and while it's a little odd having a guy touch me that much, I gotta tell you, he's got a great touch. Nice and light, deft, vaguely sensuous.

The lump was in my groin — obviously if it could have been a hernia — so he starts pushing and prodding, going back and forth, side to side, deciding what was what, and I kept thinking that if he didn't stop with that nice touch, we might have a whole other swelling problem to deal with.

But he pronounced me clear and that was all I was looking for. Evidently, Interferon can do odd things to the human body. Doc said he had a man who actually grew new lymph nodes! So now I'm waiting for a second mouth or third arm like that kid in China. Maybe another penis….

I can't begin to tell you how scared I was. Hell, I didn't tell anyone except Officer Friendly and my wife and she didn't even know until a few days after I found it. I spent the entire week thinking about shit like living wills and last wills, snapping at people, unable to sleep, unable to focus.

But even though I knew I was stressed, I didn't realize how wound up I was until he said I was clear. Then I was giddy for damn near a half hour. Everything was funny and everyone was nice and I'd laugh so hard about stupid crap I'd get teary-eyed. Yeah, no emotional high there, huh?

I remember in high school I had a cyst on my wrist. Even as someone who, at that time, was going to become a professional musician, I wasn't worried about the thing. It didn't hurt my playing so who gives a rip. Now, twenty years later with $1000 a month of chemo, any little bump or bruise or ache or pain sends me screaming to the doctor's office. I guess I've become one of those hypochondriacs I like to laugh at. On the other hand, wouldn't I rather get panicked over something that wasn't a problem, rather than ignore something that might kill me?

Uh…let me think…yes.

Yet I did have one really great moment this week.

I vandalized a local police officer's house. Hehehehehe….

For months, I had threatened to replace Ben Atkinson's American flag with my Texas flag. So Tuesday, I headed over there and was in the middle of hanging up the Texas banner when I hear: "What are you doing?"

Standing on a plastic chair, knife and string in hand, flag draped over my shoulder, I turned to the voice.

His friggin' wife! What in hell is she doing home? Maybe one chance in a million that anyone is going to be around because they both work and the kids go to daycare, and there she is! Staring at me like I've lost my mind!

"What are you doing to my house?"

"Uh…vandalizing it."

Honestly, she didn't look particularly surprised.

Then I tried desperately to switch the conversation to something else, anything else. We talked for a while, then she sighed, shook her head, and said, "Go ahead and do your vandalism, I didn't see anything."

So I hang up the flag and maybe an hour later, Ben comes banging on my front door. He had the flag semi-wadded up in his hand! A Texas flag! Threw it back at me and while he didn't laugh much, he also didn't shoot me so I guess that's a happy medium.

Then I told him about the lump and his laugh pretty much stopped. Even in every day stuff, even when I'm trying to have some fun, the beast has to roar at me, like it's worried I'll forget it's around.

But I'm trying not to dwell on that today. Today, I'm thinking about the doc's soft touch, about his pronouncement, and about the fact that I'm more than halfway home.

Holy shit, December 2 can't get here soon enough.

Comments

Catyanna, Jun 9, 2006

That's great news! Funny about the flag too.

Anonymous, Jun 9, 2006

You might have to take the hug and kiss back from Officer Friendly… wadding up our flag. That ain't fittin' it just ain't fittin. We have killed people for less much less. Since you got caught you must be slipping (damn cancer). Keep fighting the good fight. 177 days and the party will begin. I'm counting down with you.

I'm glad to hear that the doctor said everything is okay. You aren't a hypochondriac you are cautious. There is a big difference!

Grandmother Smith, Jun 10, 2006

And you thought the wind had come up strong from the south, didn't you? That was actually a big, big sigh of relief from Oklahoma!

Tammy A, Jun 10, 2006

I really didn't want to post to this, give me a heads up when we can talk. I have some stories about treatments.

Love ya and miss ya.

Anonymous, Jun 15, 2006

Glad it turned out okay!

Ellen D, Jun 17, 2006

Been out of the country since May 21st so just caught up with your blog. I'm so relieved for you Trey.

Part 33
June 23, 2006 – 11:15 am

"Trey, what are you eating?" asked Investigator DD. She sat at the second squad room table, watching me intently.

Fork to food to mouth. Fork to food to mouth.

"What are you eating?" she asked again.

I frowned. "What?"

"What. Are. You. Eating."

"Uh...I don't know. Some Mexican food thing. Some enchiladas, I think. Chicken enchiladas, Spanish rice. Why?"

"What brand is that?"

I looked at the box. "I don't know. Lean Ones, maybe?"

"It's diet food."

"Oh, okay, I guess it is."

"Diet food?"

"So what's the problem?"

"You've lost like 50 pounds," she yelled. "Why are you eating diet food?"

Hmmm, fair point. Maybe Lean Cuisine and the like aren't the best thing for me to eat. But at least I was eating, right?

At least I wasn't skipping yet another meal.

The weight is still coming off, but seems to be at a slower pace so maybe that's good. I find myself eating more frequently, just smaller amounts because too much food just makes me sick.

It's working for me right now.

In news of the strange, though, my scary lump from last week is gone. Yeah. Gone as quickly and mysteriously as it had appeared. Damn, my bid for a second penis poofed away, and having it disappear like it was never there freaked me out almost as much as its appearance had.

On the other hand, now I've got some kind of chest cold thing filling my lungs with copious amounts of phlegm. Not terrible, just enough to make my chest hurt when I try to exercise and to keep me from sleeping too well. I called my regular doctor, thinking I might get in next week.

They said "Tomorrow." Then added, don't screw around here, Trey.

It's entirely possible, they said, that if I have an infection of some kind, it could truly screw me up because my immune system is dead right now. I don't think it's that bad but when your doctor, your nurses, your wife, and your mother tell you to go, you lower your head, say "Yes, ma'am," and go.

Other than that, everything is trundling along. As usual, I'm tired, I'm cranky, I'm sure as shit tired of doctors, but everything else is as fine as it will be until December 2.

But I'm tired of getting yelled at, too. Actually, I'm tired of getting yelled at by my dear friend Investigator DD. That wasn't the first time she honked on me about food.

"Eat that," she said last week.

"But I'm not hungry."

"I don't care, eat it anyway."

"But I'm not — "

"Eat it, rookie."

I'm not really a rookie, but after two and a half years at the Sheriff's Office, I am still last on the seniority list.

'It' was a Happy Meal from McDonald's. So I ate it, and played with the tow truck car that came with it.

Ten minutes later, she wanted the car!

"You get the food, I get the car," she said.

Well, thanks a lot. I had thought she was concerned about me and wanted me to fatten up a little. Turns out I was wrong, she just wanted the car!

"Fine, take the damned car."

"It's not a car, it's Tow Mater."

"Uh...okay, whatever."

Actually, I can't bitch too much, she was the first one to take me out for food when I was able to eat again. And not only food, but barbeque.

Okay, maybe I'm not so pissed at her. But she's gotta quit saying, "Don't worry, you only have six months left."

It's not six months, it's five and a half.

Comments

Debbie B, Jun 23, 2006

You know the person that invented that has to be from Texas. Just catching up on your last few blogs. WTF is wrong with you? So glad to hear you don't have cancer...again. Real sorry to hear it's not a new "winkie" growing – that would be funny. Lost 50lbs huh? I've lost 20lbs on Weight Watchers. I know that has nothing to do with you – at least you're smiling right now and thanking someone that you were able to leave Midland.

Take care my friend.

P.S. Is Tammy "A" Tammy A- ? Hi Tammy A-, it's Debbie B-. Are you still in Midland?

Stace J, Jun 23, 2006

Add me to the list, Trey. Your doctors and loved ones are right; don't waste time wondering about the chest cold when you have no immune system. Get it checked out, pronto. In the end, it was a chest cold that did my brother in after his chemo, so don't fuck around with it. Please.

Trey, to Debbie B, Jun 24, 2006

Tomatoer...ah...I get it. That kind of sophisticated humor is sometimes beyond me. Just to answer your question, Tammy A is indeed that person. I've got her email address somewhere around.

Trey to Stace, Jun 24, 2006

I know, Stace, could be ugly. I had no idea what had happened to your brother. Trust me, I got to the doc's pretty quick. I've got a new Cancer Chronicles all about it...or will have in a few minutes anyway.

Dani D, Jun 26, 2006

I have quite a few of those tow mater trucks at my house. Want me to send you one? Of course I would have to take it from one of the Day Care kids. But hey it builds character, right?!
Take care

Part 34
June 24, 2006 – 2:07 pm

So it's nothing.

That's good, right? Blood work came back clear, chest x-ray came back clear, office tests — most of them — were clear.

All is good.

Except, it strikes me that it's not particularly good. For the last few months, I've spent quite a bit of time exercising. Three times a week, about an hour per session. I walk/jog a mile and a half, lift a few weights, do a few sit-ups. Mr. Universe it ain't, but it's been good for me.

When I started, it took me about four days to walk that mile and a half. Up until last week, my best time was just above 17 minutes. That was good, made me smile. Even in the face of chemo three times a week, I was making progress, getting slowly healthier.

But then about a week ago, my time rose to about 19 minutes. Next time out, I could only manage 1.2 miles and that hurt. Then less than a mile and then a half mile at best. And my times rose, too. From 17 to 19, then to about 20 (a 20 minute pace, I should say, because I wasn't able to actually go the full 1.5 miles)

But more than that, my chest hurt while I was doing the run. Hurt deep in my chest, not near my heart. Coughing, lots of sweat, shortness of breath. Classic signs of a heart attack I know, but I've been there and it didn't feel the same.

That's when I realized I wasn't breathing very well. On top of all the other health problems, I also have a double-deviation in my septum. In fact, that's what got the cancer-watch started. I went to get the nose fixed and the doc said he didn't want to touch me until we knew exactly what the small lump in my neck was. That was the first sign of the melanoma.

Now he won't fix my nose until the chemo is done…which I agree with…but which makes me nutty just the same.

Because sometimes I can't breathe very well. For whatever reason, right now I'm in a period where I'm not breathing well so exercising is harder. Maybe it's summer allergies or the humidity. Who knows?

But the nurse practitioner told me something, too. She reminded me that chemo builds up. Like corrosion on a car battery, I told her. She didn't care for that analogy but there you go. In other words, five minutes from now, after I take today's shot, there will be more of it in my system than there is right now. Tuesday, when I get another shot, there'll be still more.

Thursday ditto.

Yeah, yeah, yeah, I know all this, I've been through it before. But for whatever reason, I had thought we were done with that kind of thing. Apparently not.

So this is what makes me believe it isn't good that all of yesterday's tests came back clean. If there is no cold or pneumonia or whatever, then this is the new benchmark, the new standard. Chances are good I won't be able to do much better on my exercise until I'm done with the poison.

That's kind of depressing. Not hugely depressing, not like having inoperable brain cancer or needing a new heart. But vaguely depressing anyway. I had in mind where I wanted to get on my exercise and this tells me I probably won't get there until after.

Yeah, that's fine, just a mild annoyance. Kind of like dropping your ice cream cone against your shirt when you're a kid. "Well, hell, now I figure out some other way to eat this thing."

When I mentioned at the top most of the tests came back clear and good? Well, there was one that the medicos weren't happy about. My blood pressure came back 78 over 53.

Whoa, Nelly. No wonder I don't feel like doing anything but sleeping.

"You should be comatose," she said.

"Tee it up, baby," I said. "I could use with a four or five week coma right now. No responsibilities, no cares, no phone calls, no inmates. Nothing but sleep? Yeah, get to coma-ing."

Comments

Mom, Jun 25, 2006

Yep, it's still cumulative. And if you're still losing weight, that's going to affect you, too. Be super glad you were in top shape to start all this. And you will be again, too – just not next Tuesday.

Part 35
Thursday. June 29th, 2006

So, after two weeks of worsening times on my little 1.5 mile walk/jog, after two weeks of not being able to finish the distance, of not being able to breathe, of having a few painful coughs from deep in my chest, I did pretty well yesterday.

Nearly 2 miles on an 18 minute pace. Hurt, but I got through it.

WTF?

It is official, I have no idea what chemo is doing to me. Some days it's terrible, some days not so bad, and some days are almost like regular days. No consistency.

Whatever.

I think I mentioned a while back about giving myself shots exclusively in my stomach. Well, the endless shots and taking a while to heal had left me with a stomach riddled with holes and scabs and everything else.

So I went to the hospital to talk to Tamara about it. She laughed and said, "You know you can give the shots elsewhere."

Uh…no, hadn't known that.

Put them in your arm or your butt or your thigh, anywhere you can pinch up some skin.

Great, I thought. And it's been fabulous. I rotate, right thigh then left thigh then abdomen, then back again. Nothing ever gets too beat up.

But here's what I realized a few nights ago when I took a shot at the jail: I've lost so much weight in my thighs that I didn't have to lower my trousers. I was able just to pull my pants leg up, damn near to my hip, and do the shot. How freakishly weird is that?

Just another of those bizarre details.

A few days ago, a friend said something about only having six months left of chemo. I got a little cranky.

"Fuck that," I said. "Five and a half months! Don't charge me for the extra two weeks."

At the time, I remember thinking: how so very childish. Like a kid you ask how old he is and he says "Six and a half," or "Five and three-quarters," or whatever.

Childish childish childish.

But here I am on June 28 and I keep thinking, "Five months and four days!"

Not that I'm counting, of course.

That would be childish.

Part 36
Tuesday, July 4th, 2006

Okay, not that I'm obsessing about the days left on chemo treatment, but I'm now officially less than 5 months left.

Wheee-haawwww!

Strange to think it's been seven months since all this bullshit started. What's more strange is that some of it — going to the treatment room, trying to sleep or read during the daily treatments, being hesitant and scared when it came time to give my first shots myself — seems like a bad dream. It's kind of soft and fuzzy, like bad photos in a late '70's Penthouse magazine.

Here's an odd detail. I've complained to people about my mouth, how it always feel coated and thick and nasty. I was sitting outside this morning, playing ball with the dogs, and I spit. What hit the sidewalk was solid white and didn't evaporate in the heat.

Ooooohhhh, gimme some more of that.

No wonder everything has an aftertaste, huh?

But only five months left. Five months five months five months. Call it my new mantra. Some people have "Ohhhhmmmmmm," I have five months left.

Good news on another front, too. A writer friend of mine, battling cancer far worse than mine, and battling it longer than I have been, just got back from the Mayo clinic. He went to see about a transplant. The doctors did some work, discovered things were slightly better than everyone had thought, and put the transplant off for a while.

I wish him all the best and for those of you who've said you're praying for me, toss some prayers his way. He needs them, too.

Part 37: News Good Bad Ugly
July 13, 2006 – 3:19 pm

It's hard to explain how much I hate all this.

I find it difficult to dig up the right words, to make myself clear. Maybe I'm just a shitty writer, but maybe it's because chemo keeps me generally foggy and muddy-brained.

Regardless of the why, the right words just won't come.

Maybe some of the details will help. Most nights, I'm in bed about ten hours. It'd be great if all that were sleep, but it's not. Quite a few nights I only sleep for tiny snatches of time stuffed in between periods of being wide awake. All this in spite of wanting to sleep 24 hours a day. When I do wake up in the mornings I know — with absolute certainty — I'll be tired all day or have a headache all day or be unable to eat. That knowledge is wearing.

Most days, I find myself sitting in my office or in the squad room at work or behind the counter at the bookstore with my head in my hands, my stomach roiling around while my legs and feet become heavy as clay. There is simply no energy to do whatever needs to be done.

As a writer, I tend to write pretty fast; couple of chapters per week. But with the new novel, I've done four chapters in six months. There is simply no motivation, even though I love where I am so far, to go work on the damned thing.

Who knows why I'm writing all this, I've gone through it before, over and over until I'm sure you're as sick of reading about it as I am of writing about it. But what's different, what has surprised me, is that I'd thought it would be great once I got better than halfway done.

It's not great, it's the same old drudgery. The tyranny of routine, I guess.

At the doctor this morning, Dr. Vukov was happy with most of the tests — blood work, chest x-ray, physical, etc — and said all my levels looked good and normal...normal for where I am, anyway. But he was concerned about my x-ray from a couple weeks ago.

"You've got a slightly enlarged heart," he said.

Holy fucking crap.

He tried to assure me it was probably nothing, that Interferon does all kinds of strange things (and told me a story of a patient of his having massive kidney failure...uh, thanks, Doc, that picks me right up) but that once I'm done with the treatment, all that will fade back to normal.

Maybe it's the chemo, maybe it's a gathering of fluid around the heart. Maybe this maybe that blah blah blah.

Then he asked me about any history of heart disease in my family. "Uh, yeah. Grandfather dead at 30 of a heart attack, father had a heart attack at 32. Mine was at 34. So, yeah, bit of a history there."

Between that and telling him that I have a bit of shortness of breath when I exercise (maybe it's because of the double-deviation in my septum...maybe it's because of the unremitting humidity the last few weeks...maybe it's because of allergies...maybe this maybe that blah blah blah) I'm suddenly scheduled for an echogram and some kind of breathing test.

And oddly, I'm not worried about the tests (I think it's the chemo's fault), but I'm worried about how the hell I'm going to pay for all this crap. The bills have piled and piled until the hospital asked me if I wanted either a low-interest loan to get them paid off or an application to be classified as a charity case. In other words, go deeper into debt to pay the debt or be pathetic.

Thanks, I appreciate it.

Mostly, at this point, I just want a break. I want a two or three week break with no drugs and no tests and no inmates and no phone calls and no jobs. A medical furlough, I guess.

Sadly, not going to happen.

But, in a bit of decent news, the doctor has agreed to give me another break from the chemo. A week, anytime in the next few days, and then when I get back on, he might lower the dosage just a bit.

Not as much as I wanted, but more than I thought I'd get. I'll take it.

And in the ugly news, yet another family member died recently.

My Uncle Bud Hamilton. I didn't know him well but enjoyed his company whenever I found myself in it. Though he'd been sick in the past, he'd been fairly healthy lately. His death wasn't as much of a shock as with William, but shocking none the less. Because of my general weakness, I won't be able to drive the sixteen hours to go to his funeral.

Man, oh, man, I need a break.

December 2...december 2...december 2....

Comments

Grandmother Smith, Jul 15, 2006

Trey, I just returned from Bud's funeral which was yesterday. He was a great person – the kind who held everything together and helped wherever he could. I think you'll be pleased to know that the last song sung at his funeral was one Bud hummed whenever he got in his car to take a trip: Willie's "On the Road Again". The family all thought of you when we were together and wished you well.

Part 38: It's Like So Many Things
July 17, 2006 – 5:11 pm

Aaahhhhhhhhhh….

It's like so many things, this being off the chemo for a week. It's like the afterglow of really great sex. It's like the perfect ice cream cone when the temperature outside is sweaty-hot, but not instantly-melting-your-cone hot. It's like the perfect spring morning in the mountains when birds different from the ones heard in the city sing.

Mostly, it's like having the black hood taken off my head. Suddenly, I can see again. Suddenly, I can breathe again.

Suddenly I've got energy and an appetite and my jokes are funny again…okay, semi-funny.

What has been interesting to me, during this particular break, is the self-awareness of the depression. I knew, last week, I was depressed. I knew it was probably mostly chemo-induced, with touches of concern about my enlarged heart, about the last four months to go, about my exercise routine, etc.

This is going to be tough to explain so bear with me (and yes, those of you dying in this massive heat sink with no air conditioning can bare with me).

Intellectually, I knew — or was pretty sure, anyway — the depression and all of its effects were from the chemo. I believed I ought to be able to ignore it. If I know my life in general wasn't the source, then I should be able to compartmentalize, to say, "I know what this is and it's not me so piss off."

But I couldn't. Even as I sank further into depression, even as I knew what was causing it, I couldn't stop it. And trust me, it was deeper than it's ever been, stronger and more pervasive. Maybe that's because I had the enlarged heart hanging over me, too, I don't know. But this time, the depression scared the shit outta me.

Now, four days since my last injection, I'm fucking rocking, dudes and dudettes. Sgt. Atkinson even bemoaned his vacation schedule today, "I've got four days of you like this before I can leave the state," or words to that effect.

'Like this' is energy-ridden, bouncing off the walls, singing pirate songs ("I am a swashbuckling pirate man. With a giant righteous gland and sword as big as a ship." It's my own creation, thank you, very much.), telling great jokes, being a general pain in the ass.

The depression lifted that easily, that quickly, and left me doing this odd navel-gazing analysis of the problem, of how self involved it was to think about the whole thing. It reminded me of that really great scene in *Ocean's Twelve* where Julie Roberts, playing Tess, agrees to Tess' impersonating Julia Roberts and then calls Roberts' house, only to talk to…the 'real' Julia Roberts. I know, a tenuous connection at best. But I think of it because of what thinking about the depression and its cause does to my brain. I know what it is so I shouldn't think about it but I can't because it scares me because maybe it's not totally the chemo even while I know that when I'm off the chemo it won't exist anymore blah blah blah.

Anyway, right now, today, I'm not even depressed about the time I have left on the juice. I'll juice up again later this week, maybe this weekend, and I'll go a couple of months, then take another little break for a writers convention, then be done a few weeks after that.

Last week, I was ready to blow my fuggin' brains out because of four and a half months left. Today, hey, it's what has to be done. That simple, that easy to digest. This is where I am, fair or not, do what I gotta do.

Can you tell I feel good? Hell, I'm writing my brains out on this damn journal and it's not even all that interesting.

Hah, check back next week. I'll be cranky and tired and depressed and moaning about the state of the world.

Yeah, can't wait for that.

Comments

Scanner Darkly, Jul 17, 2006

It's good to see you cheery. Even if it's possibly temporary. It still kicks ass.

Keep on keepin' on, man.

Amy K, Jul 18, 2006

I'm saying this with all the love in my heart... Suck it up!

Be cranky if you need to. Take the good days when they come and be grateful when you have them. You know the bad days will come but they also go. You have come so far and yes, depression is part of it. They are POISONING your body and you are beating the hell out of cancer. Who wouldn't get down a little.

I'm proud that you keep writing and keeping me posted. I look forward to each entry even if you are cranky. I would love to hear a "Live" version of the pirate song.

Keep up the good fight and by my calculations 138 more days. I could be off a day or two... I'm sure you will let me know if I am.

Part 39
July 23, 2006 – 4:32 pm

What a week!

Eating like a pig, exercising going extremely well, sleep doing okay, tons of energy, tons of really hy-sterical jokes. What a great week.

Sadly, tonight I'll go back on the juice. I hate that, but the doctor decided we'll lower the dosage again and see how things do. So I'll go from 16 million units to 14 million. Last time he lowered the dosage, the result was like, as Steve Martin says, "discovering verbs...my novels really brightened up after that."

Not much to say this time around. Everything is great and I love life again. Got some good writing done this week, got some good housework done this week.

Oh, stupid ass, almost forgot. I went to the hospital Tuesday and had some tests. The Doc was concerned about pain in my chest when I exercise, shortness of breath, and a slightly enlarged heart.

So I did the echocardiogram, which is like an ultrasound. The tech wouldn't comment officially but said she'd been doing it awhile and didn't see any problems. Then I went to the breathing test, convinced I had just about zero lung capacity. Well, turns out I was WAAAAAAAYYYY higher than the averages. Every test came up 109, 111, 113, 119 percent higher than normal. The breathing tech said that had nothing to do with any deviated septum, just lung capacity.

Anyway, the doc said both tests looked good. He's convinced the enlargement is from the chemo, believes it'll go away pretty quickly after I get off the chemo. So that was good news, and seemed to be borne out by the fact that only a week off the juice, my exercising was the best I've ever done.

I did have an interesting thought, though. Talking to my mama yesterday (after she 'voiced concern' about my exercising too much. I love her but she'll always be the mama, you know?), she told me it turns out my uncle Bud died of leukemia. No one even knew he had it and it wasn't apparent until after the blood work got back days after he was dead.

A person's normal white blood cell count is between 4,500 and 10,000. Uncle Bud's was 42,000.

Holy White Blood, Batman!

Mom said the white blood cells were generating new white blood cells so fast that his red blood cells were getting squeezed out. Red blood cells, as we all know, carry oxygen to the organs and limbs and where ever. So his system was losing oxygen. The organ shut down was so fast that even though he was in the hospital by midnight, he was dead by 8 a.m.

There were no other symptoms of the cancer.

Man, how scary is that?

Anyway, that got me to wondering. Are my oxygen problems — breathing during exercise — vaguely related to that? I know my red blood cell count is down a bit, though I'm not sure how much. Could it be that my systems aren't getting enough oxygen when I push them a bit harder?

I wonder, too, if suddenly hitting the wall on the exercise a few weeks ago was where the oxygen depletion was. In other words, I did fine for a long while because I hadn't hit the limit of oxygen in my blood yet; I still had room to improve. But I've improved so much now that maybe this is the best I can do until I'm off the juice.

Maybe that's it...coupled with the juice, too, obviously.

Idle speculation. Doesn't matter anyway. I'll do what I can do, keep exercising because it helps me feel better (the endorphin rush is very cool) and because it helps my immune system. When I'm done with the poison, I'll do better.

Actually, I feel pretty good about it all right now. It'll be interesting to see if I still feel this good by mid-week when I'm taking the shots again. That depression that I know is chemo-induced but that I can't seem to do anything about might be back.

Piss on it.

Amy K had it right a few days ago in her comments.

"Suck it up," she said. "By my calculation (it's) 138 more days."

Actually, right now, it's down to 132 days, with one more little break end of September. It's getting close…so close. Maybe I'll start posting every day when I'm down to 100, just a constant daily countdown. Like a VH1 special: The 100 Greatest Days Until Chemo Free Countdown.

Shit, I should submit that, maybe make some money, help pay for the chemo.

Comments

Mama, Jul 24, 2006

Yep, you're right, Kiddo. I'll always be the mama. Can't help it – it's in the job description. And you know I *always* take my jobs seriously.

Part 40
Monday, July 31st, 2006

Wow, who'd have thought I'd write 40 damn installments of this crap?

Of course, there were times when I never thought I'd be this close to being done, either. Four months…124 days.

Wheee-haaawwww.

So I've been on the lowered dosage for about a week. Overall, it seems to be better. I'm less fatigued, less weak, less cranky. I still have all those symptoms, but they're not quite as bad.

Still, the biggest consistency is the inconsistency. One day a shot doesn't bother me at all, the next day it leaves me sleeping for 18 hours and stumbling around like a drunk.

What the hell is that? I get all the drawbacks of being drunk and none of the advantages. That bites.

Anyway, not much to write about this go-round.

Maybe not having anything to say right now is good. Means there have been no truly terrible days, no trips to the hospital, nothing like that.

On the other hand, maybe not having anything to say is bad. Means it's all become so routine, so daily, that I hardly notice it anymore.

Way back in December, when all this started, it took me a while to get used to 'cancer victim,' or 'cancer patient,' or whatever. I simply couldn't get my head around having that attached to my name.

Now, it appears I have a whole new thing to get used to: 'cancer survivor,' or 'kicked cancer's ass long and hard and then spit on it.'

Again, a strange thing to hear after your name, but more cool than what I was hearing in December.

Part 44: Something Different
August 1, 2006 – 12:08 pm

There is a writer whose work I've always loved. He has the ability to put me so deeply inside a crackling good story that hours fly by uncounted.

Since my battle with cancer started, he has been amazingly supportive. Because he, too, has cancer.

When I talked with him recently, I asked if he'd be interested in writing a piece for the *Cancer Chronicles*. His experience with C is vastly different — and will continue to be vastly different — than mine. I thought it would be interesting to get a taste of what he goes through.

So here it is.

Two weeks ago I lost my innocence…
by Ed Gorman

For the past five years I've had multiple myeloma, an incurable but treatable cancer that works like termites in wood. MM eats the marrow of your bones until your bones collapse.

In some cases, people with MM die soon after diagnosis. Others live, on average, around 5-7 years. In my case I wasn't even treated for the disease until I'd had it for five years. This is called "smoldering" mm. In other words, there's smoke but no fire. Yes, I had symptoms, sometimes so painful that I had to use a cane to walk across the room. But I was never given any cancer drugs.

We all have appreciation for things in the abstract. I can imagine what it's like to be black, handsome, rich. I have enough of an imagination that I can even flesh these other-lives out to some degree.

So it was with cancer drugs. When you have cancer you generally get to know a whole lot of other cancer victims. Makes sense. You see each other at the oncologist's if nowhere else.

And of course you TALK about cancer and the treatments attendant on such. You even see the results of the treatments on your fellow sufferers–the pale flesh, the weight loss, the hair loss, the sadness, the fear.

I saw all these things in my friends and tried to prepare myself for the inevitable day when I'd become full-blown mm and would require the drugs that were taking such a toll on those around me. I even IMAGINED myself taking them, dealing with them.

Take my word for it, imagination has severe limitations. Two weeks ago I was put on four cancer drugs and my life changed instantly and profoundly. Among the worst symptoms have been memory loss, confusion, dizziness that has knocked me to my knees, nausea, savage heart rate, color-blips in my peripheral vision and depression added to the depression I've suffered all my life.

And I'm not even taking the dreaded chemo, chemo not working for mm.

Right now I've got two friends who are battling for their lives, trying to survive chemo regimens that just might (and I'm serious here) make me roll over and die rather than try to get through it. I pray for them several times a day. There's not much else I can do.

This is just FYI for all you innocent of cancer in your lives. That old cliche about the cure sometimes being worse than the disease? We all want to live and thanks to modern medicine most of will live longer than we would have even ten years ago. But there's a price to be paid for survival. So next time a friend of yours says he or she has cancer, lavish them with hearty good wishes. That's still the best medicine of all, especially since some people still run from you when they know you have cancer.

Comments

John P, Aug 1, 2006
Amen.

Part 42: Just A Few Stitches....
August 19, 2006 – 2:55 pm

Back in 2001, when I had my heart attack, a number of friends came to me, faces white with fear, their big bellies quivering.

"That scared the shit outta me," most of them said.

"Uh…yeah…me, too," I answered.

"I'm gonna get in shape," they said. "You know, eating better, getting some exercise, taking better care of myself."

Believe it or not, some of them did. One writer friend of mine, known for his incredible short stories, did lose some weight, did take better care of himself.

So I felt like I had helped, like maybe I had done something good for my friends.

A few days ago, a Princeton Police sergeant (not Officer Friendly), stopped me in the street.

"I want to thank you for saving my life," he said.

"Uh…yeah…sure."

He showed me his forearm. A neat pink scar stared back at me. Seems he noticed a new spot some days before. He went to the doctor, they cut it off, stitched up the hole, and tested the lump.

It came back pre-cancerous.

He had the spot looked at, he said, because of what I've gone through.

Yeah? Well, good then.

It is the same sentiment I had after the heart attack, after so many people let me know it was damned lucky for them the heart attack was mine. My suffering, they all implied, really saved them some grief.

And I don't mean to be shitty or selfish. I mean it sincerely. I look at it this way: I would have suffered the heart attack and the cancer regardless, so if my friends can get something good out of it all, that might be the best of all possible newses (or the best of all possible worlds...and I'll send some cool free gift to whoever can name that reference.)

I won't go so far as to say I saved any lives, but I will take credit for raising some awareness.

I am at about three and a half months left of chemo now. Getting closer and closer and that's a good thing, but the closer I get, the worse it gets for me mentally. It's short-timer's disease.

Like the last few days of a job or, as the inmates at my jail constantly tell me, the last few hours of a jail sentence. I get more and more antsy as the days pass.

Otherwise, I'm doing well enough right now; just about the same number of bad days as good...and that's a pretty good step forward.

You can tell I generally feel decent because I haven't written in a few days. I seem to write more when I'm pissy and tired and hurting. Maybe when I feel better, I want to do things I haven't been able to do much this year.

I have been incredibly tired the last few weeks. I've worked overnights at the jail and it's tough to coordinate that with the shots. So I spend more of my shift tired than when I work day shift.

Anyway, I took the week off from chemo a couple weeks ago and it was great. Then I got back on at a slightly lower dosage. One good thing: I can eat better than before. One bad thing: my depth perception is strangely off.

Can't tell you how many times I've walked into a wall or door or desk or something.

I'm not worried about it. Rather, I find myself doing strange little eye experiments, just kind of exploring this twist in my vision. I've always had perfect vision and hearing (in spite of twenty plus years of drums and guitars and Drum Corps and whatnot) so it's interesting to see what things are like for people with eyes less than perfect.

So something good came out of the cancer. Given everything I've been through — what a pain in the balls this whole thing has been — I'll take the Sergeant's good news.

And when he gets around to buying me a Corona or two, I'll take that, too.

Comments

Anonymous, Aug 22, 2006

"The best of all possible worlds" is from "Candide" (Voltaire). Send a donation to your local animal shelter.

Part 43: Breaking 100
August 26, 2006 – 12:52 pm

99 and counting....

Comments

Mom, Aug 27, 2006
Hooray! You broke 100!

Part 44: Something Different
September 1, 2006 – 8:47 pm

So, I've started this entry about 40 hundred times and nothing works. Can't seem to write my way out of an old wino's paperbag.

Damn writer's block. I'm sure it's the chemo's fault.

Okay, less chemo than general stupidity but there it is.

But part of it, too, is that there simply isn't much to write about right now. Yes, I'm tired. Yes, I have days of crankiness (ain't that a movie? Days of Whine and Crankiness?). Yes, I still don't eat much. But I've written about all that before, you've read about all that before. Right now, it's the same old thing. To a lesser degree, but still the same old thing.

Honestly, I'm getting friggin' sick and tired of the same old thing. But better days are coming. And here's how I know that: a few nights ago, LuAnn asked me to make up some of my enchiladas. I haven't done that for nearly a year because they tasted awful and I wasn't hungry anyway.

She loves 'em so I made 'em up because she asked.

And then I promptly sucked up two like they were free Corona beer. And wanted two more!

Holy Chalupa, Batman!

They hit the spot in a way absolutely no food has done for nearly a year. That's a good sign. Hell, that's a great sign.

The other way I know things are getting better is that I don't find myself fighting through the massive depression both the chemo and being a cancer victim brought with it. I still get agitated and angry, but I don't often find myself sitting around depressed about it all. Sure, it still happens, but how often it happens, and the degree to which it hits me, is less than it was.

That, damn near in and of itself, makes me feel like the light at the end of the tunnel is getting larger.

So, here's what I thought I'd do, just to keep everything interesting. A few weeks ago, I had Ed Gorman write a piece about living with cancer. It occurred to me then that my cancer doesn't affect just me, but everyone around me. Yeah, yeah, an obvious realization, so I'll blame chemo-brain for not having it earlier.

The cancer touches LuAnn and my mom and family and friends on the force and writer friends and casual friends. In one way or another, it touches a great many people. So I asked a couple of them to write a little about the entire thing. And yeah, I realize that's mostly ego — how does MY cancer affect how you deal with ME? — but I thought it'd be interesting anyway.
In the next entry, probably later tonight, I'll have something from my mother. I hope you enjoy it. If you don't, I'll send you some of my enchiladas…assuming I haven't eaten them all.

Comments

Kylie, Sep 2, 2006

Hi. I've been reading you posts for a long time now. It never ceases to amaze me how brutally honest you are with yourself and how mortal we all are, yet there is such grace and humour in your words. Makes me ashamed to whine about having a shitty day. Hypoglycaemia is NOTHING compared to you.

And I have survived my own battle with cancer. I was lucky, it was caught in time. And even so I forget how scary that was because its (mostly) over. Sure, it inspired me to develop myself and do the things I live for a living but sometimes its too easy to forget that as a decently healthy person, I've got nothing to complain about.

Me…see there I go again. I was wanting to praise you. To thank you, for sharing this, your words, pain, humour and honesty with all of us. I notice you never get comments but I'm sure that many of us read your words with wrapt awe. You are my inspiration. Those days when I feel hard done by, or that life is unfair, I remember my past fight with cancer, and I remember you. And you remind me that even in the hardest times, there are still so many ways to see humour, to process pain, and to reach out to others with humility and grace.

Thank you.

Part 45: I'm The Mama
Friday, September 1st, 2006

My Son's Mortality
by Alison Evans

When Trey was a kid (age 34), his wife called me at our Trading Post and told me he was in the hospital and had suffered a heart attack. I asked her if this was some kind of bad joke. Trey is known for those. No such luck. Scared the peewaddley out of me.

Here's the horrible part of being a mom. I am biased about my kids. Always have been, I guess. Any truly honest parent will admit to this failing. Well, hey – this one practically raised himself with nary a whine, whimper or teenage rebellion. No wonder he impressed me so much. So the first thing I thought was that I was going to lose one of my sons early in life – probably in retribution for my multitude of sins. No kidding, that was my thought process.

After that, Trey did well at his recovery and I slowly got over my fears. Case closed, right?

Again, no such luck. Now the kid was age 39 – still almost a babe. The removal of the lymph node didn't worry me until the diagnosis came back. Now I'm scared shitless again. Am I still sinning so badly that the Great Beyond has it in for me? What? ME? Aren't I supposed to be worrying about Trey?

And I did. As soon as the Interferon started hitting him and he started suffering the effects of it.

There is nothing so hard as to watch your own child suffer and not be able to do anything about it. A minor example: when Trey was 10 years old, he talked the Powers That Be at the Midland Reporter-Telegram into letting him be a paper carrier a year earlier than was their normal procedure. On his first day of throwing papers, I was driving home from work and happened to see him on his bike trying to haul all those papers and having a really hard time of it. I could have taken part of his load and done it for him. But I didn't. I made him finish the route, then when he got home, we figured out an easier way for him to split the load from then on. But leaving him there in the middle of the street, struggling with that load, was one of the hardest things I've ever had to do. I cried all the way home.

Now, with the Interferon, there is no way I can even offer to take part of the load. So now all I can do is worry, pray, joke with him and be there for dumping purposes. And it hurts so badly that I can't carry that load.

So now I check his blog daily, hoping for news – even if it's bad. And I count down the days as avidly as he does. And I wish over and over that I could be the one suffering.

Part 46
Monday, September 11th, 2006

Those damned white blood cells. It's like they've got a mind of their own. "Hey, I know what'll be fun," I can hear them saying, "Now that things are going so well for ol' Trey, let's take a nose dive and see what happens."

Went to the doctor last week and everything — save the white blood cell count — was good. Doctor actually was sort of bored. But for whatever reason, and he had no idea other than 'chemo does that sometimes,' my white blood cells are down.

Still within the range of acceptable, the doc said, but lower than they've been since I was doing the daily crap back in December.

"Don't catch a cold," he said. "Could kill you."

Uh…yeah, thanks Doc. How much am I paying you again?

So that was a little unnerving. Not quite as unnerving as finding a lump or discovering my heart was enlarged, but still….'chemo does that sometimes.'

***

In case you missed it, here are the highlights of a story that ran on *ABC News.com* a few days ago.

"Aug. 31, 2006 — Seven years ago, Mark Origer was diagnosed with a malignant melanoma, a sometimes curable skin cancer that can be deadly if it spreads to other parts of the body. By 2004, his cancer had spread to his liver, lung and lymph nodes.

"Desperate for a cure, Origer enrolled in a clinical trial at the National Cancer Institute in Bethesda, Md. The trial tested a very experimental therapy that had never before been used in people. The cancer institute's researchers are using genetically engineered immune cells to shrink tumors in cancer patients like Origer.

"This is the first gene therapy for cancer. … That is why it is so important," said Dr. Steven A. Rosenberg, who headed the trial as chief of surgery at the National Cancer Institute. Researchers took immune system cells from the blood of 17 advanced melanoma patients who, like Origer, had not been helped by conventional treatments. Origer had only three months to four months left to live when the experimental treatment began.

These ordinary blood cells, called T cells, were genetically engineered to become cancer-fighting cells that could recognize and attack the life-threatening melanoma. The cancer-fighting cells were then injected back into each patient. Researchers hoped that the new T cells would multiply and fight off the cancers."

Not only did the guy live, there isn't a drop of cancer left in his body. In other words, he's cured and he didn't have to go to Mexico, have leeches attached to his balls while he spun around four times singing *Ave Maria* and handing over his AmEx card.

Very exciting. That guy's cancer is my cancer. What started as skin cancer spread to his lymph nodes. That is what I went through. Obviously, his was much worse, much scarier. But now he's cured. Now he's safe and alive and all the rest. Part of my new reality — new since I got the diagnosis last November — is that it will come back someday. Maybe next week, maybe next month, maybe not until way down the road. But I do believe I will get cancer again at some point, and stories like this give me some hope that, while I may get it again, it probably won't kill me.

And yeah, I fully understand that something like 90 percent of the people in the study died anyway, that the therapy didn't work for them, but there is that shred of self-involved hope, isn't there? People may die, but not me, I'll be the one person for whom it works.

***

From a letter posted by a reader — Kylie — a few days ago:

"Hi. I've been reading your posts for a long time now. It never ceases to amaze me how brutally honest you are with yourself and how mortal we all are, yet there is such grace and humour in your words. Makes me ashamed to whine about having a shitty day. Hypoglycaemia is NOTHING compared to you."

It was a touching letter and I'm glad she wrote it, but it tickled something in my brain. Even at its worst, I found myself thinking, this is pretty small stuff. Compared to people with brain cancer and lung cancer and a seemingly endless string of cancer types, compared to people who had months or weeks or even days left, mine seemed pretty minor.

It sometimes seemed too petty to bitch about, in other words.

And yet, here is this woman, who's been silently reading the installments, who has battled her own cancer and now lives with other health problems that affect her damn near daily (from the sound of it) and she says the same thing about me. Why bitch about my own situation when there are other, worse situations out there?

Exactly. Though my ego would never let me not write about it, that thought has been in the back of my addled brain since this started. What the fuck am I writing for? What do I think I have to say? I can't compare to people who are looking at coffins or who are strapped down in a hospital room for days and weeks and months.

"...but sometimes," she wrote, "It's too easy to forget that as a decently healthy person, I've got nothing to complain about."

Hah! If you've got nothing to complain about, you're just not trying hard enough. (Thank you, very much, ladies and gentlemen, I'll be here all week and don't forget to tip your waitress)

Seriously, that's how I feel sometimes. Come on, Trey, this has been pretty minor, you're alive, you're healthier now than you've been in years (thanks to the Chemo Diet Plan and some exercise). What's the problem?

There is always something else further up the line that puts everything in perspective, I guess. Regardless of how bad it is, there are people hurting much worse.

Part 47
Monday, September 11th, 2006

Eight-two days....

Part 48: Feeling Groovy
September 26, 2006 – 10:37 am

"Trey?"

"Hey, Trey? Where are you?"

Exercise room. Squad room.

"Trey? You here? Trey. Hey!"

Break room. Class room. Holding cells.

"Hey. Trey! You okay? Where are you?"

Sally port. Sergeants' office. DARE office. Exercise room again.

"Trey! Damnit, don't screw with me! Where are you?"

Lobby. Hallways. Behind the exercise equipment. Bathrooms. Call the bookstore. Call the Sheriff's Office. Call my home.

And Sergeant Terry Polhemus' heart rate kept climbing.

Finally, he called Sgt. Atkinson.

"Hey, I can't find Trey. His stuff is at Post 40. He was exercising. I can't find him."

Atkinson — Officer Friendly — glanced at me. We were on an accident call together. "Uh…he's with me."

I'm not sure what Polhemus' words were after that, but I'm pretty sure they were colorful and probably included images of impaling me on the treadmill.

I didn't even think about leaving my stuff there, and maybe that's the most distressing part of the entire — now funny — incident.

When I got done with the daily poisoning in December, I realized I had lost a great majority of my muscle mass. I had trouble, in other words, doing basic things like lifting meals at the jail or holding up whatever book I was reading.

So I began to exercise. A little weight lifting, a little running. Just trying to stay as healthy as possible through all this, trying to boost my immune system. Hell, even trying to find something to keep my mind off of being sick.

And through it all, there always seemed to be one of the boys in blue around. Making jokes and always just in earshot, listening for me falling down, passing out, or dying.

(Hah, wouldn't that have been the funniest joke. I die and THEY get stuck with filling out all the paperwork and reports and insurance forms. Hah, bury them in paper!)

The point — please God make the point already, you rambling, bloviating fool — is that I wasn't worried about leaving my stuff sitting on that table. It didn't occur to me that Terry would see my keys and not my body and get worried.

In other words, I forgot he might be worried about me.

I felt that good, that healthy and strong and in control.

What the fuck? When was the last time that happened? Honestly, last October and November, when I was out shilling for my first novel. Then, in November, the Terrible Times started.

I wrote a few months ago that I had no good days. All of them were bad. Then, later, I wrote that I was having good days but they were few and far between.

Well, the ratio is changing. Call it 50/50 now. At least as many good days as bad.

Not only can I see the light at the end of the tunnel, but there's enough light now that it's warming me up pretty good. Hell, maybe even enough light to tan my face a little.

Of course, I might feel great today simply because it's sun-shiny outside, I'm on vacation from the jail for eight days, and I'm on a week's break from the poison.

Plus, this week is Bouchercon, the mystery/crime convention, and I'm looking forward to seeing some writer friends, people who've managed to help me get through the bullshit by sending me free books and stuff.

I mean, yeah, their friendship is great blah blah blah, but send me loot, man, that's what I'm all about.

By the by, 65 days....

Comments

Glen K, Sep 26, 2006

65 days. Man, that's nothing. Keep it up. Great to hear the good days are increasing.

Part 49: The Non-Memorial Shot
October 4, 2006 – 12:11 pm

The bar was dark, a band playing in the background except they were so loud it was more foreground than anything. Bodies packed tightly into the joint like crack rocks in an Altoid's tin. Smell of booze and piss and stale sweat and pheromones.

And all I saw was the amber. Four splashes of it. Beautiful, life-sustaining, arousing Jack Daniel's' amber.

"Time for a non-memorial shot," they said.

"Non-memorial of what?" I asked.

Writers Sean Doolittle, Jeff Shelby, and Lori Armstrong.

And me. Sitting in the stinking bar, crowded by body parts that we were pretty sure we didn't want to touch, crowded by lame-ass conversations, by sex-trollers, by pompous, pretentious, bloviating writers and drinkers.

"To the fact that you're not dead," one of them said.

And when it went down, when I got the first taste of whiskey since all this started last November, when I got that soft, soothing burn, I'm pretty sure I was pitching a tent.

Don't get me wrong, I don't drink a ton, but I do love the taste of Daniel's. And I hadn't had anything since we started the chemo. Some people said it wouldn't be a problem to drink while getting the poison, some said it would. Beyond the medical, there was the financial. I'm paying so much to doctors and procedures and chemo juice that I couldn't afford it anyway.

And by the by, I'm not sure who paid for the shots, but I do appreciate it!

It was that way all weekend, at the Madison, WI Bouchercon. Bouchercon is a mystery convention for writers/editors/fans/readers/agents/etc. Anyone who loves crime and mysteries.

It was an incredible weekend, punctuated by a gratifyingly high number of kisses from women saying "Oh, Trey, I'm glad you're not dead!".

Uh...me, too.

I met some incredible people over the weekend and most of them had a cancer story of their own, either themselves or someone dear to them. Listening to those stories — a woman's sister who had colon cancer for the third time and maybe she'd make it to next month and maybe she wouldn't — made me realize how large the cancer community is.

There were a couple of people who I would never have spent time with. Don't like their politics, don't like their books, don't like them, whatever. But when cancer came up, all the rest of that shit was out the window.

For that moment, it was like the *Lethal Weapon* movie where Gibson and Rene Russo compare scars. My cancer was this while his was that; my treatment was this way while hers was that.

While we talked and joked about the cancer — Sandy Loper-Herzog and John Purcell and myself using "You know (I)(he's) dying of cancer!'" — it never defined me, even during those conversations with people I wouldn't normally have talked to. We talked about the disease, but we all understood there was so much more to each story than just the disease.

In fact, I had more people talk to me about the book and the short stories and how I did what I did and how I managed the creative process and did I meet that editor or that writer or where were we going for dinner or boxers or briefs, Corona or Corona Light. The cancer was something we could all talk about, but it wasn't the only thing we could talk about.

Part of me had nervously expected otherwise.

With my close friends, obviously, I'd expected other conversations, but for those writers I was just getting to know or had met the previous year, I was worried it would be about the cancer.

I wanted people, in a nearly petulant school kid kind of way, to talk about my writing and my career and whatever. In other words, I wanted to be noticed for something other than being sick.

When I was in second or third grade, I snatched some money from Mama's purse. Anson Jones Elementary was selling these little First Aid kits as some kind of fundraiser (I think). Vinyl folding cover, stuffed with Band-Aids, antiseptic cream, little scissors, gauze wrap, aspirins.

Desperately, I wanted one of those. And as soon as I got it, I was 'Da Man. Kids would go running around, 'fall,' and need medical attention. I handed it out like fucking Dr. Kildare.

I was noticed. I was respected. More importantly, to both the second grader and the adult writer, I was the center of attention.

Here's the thing: I still wanted to be the center of attention at Bouchercon, but not for medical reasons, for arty reasons.

All writers, regardless of how shy they might be, want to be that center of attention, want the world to hear what they have to say (otherwise they probably wouldn't write for publication, right?). That was what I wanted, to stand in a conversation with people like Ken Bruen and talk about what brought us all together.

Not that Ken didn't yell at me about keeping my health up. Actually, to be brutally honest, he sort of vaguely threatened me. I take seriously anything that sounds even remotely like a threat from an Irish man who was a security guard at WTC and spent time in a Brazilian prison for a bar fight. (And can you imagine the fight that would land you in jail in Brazil? Holy crap.)

On Friday, Lori Armstrong and I went to go shoot handguns. A few of her friends went with us, people I like to think of as friends of mine now: Jeff Shelby, Alison Gaylin, Karen Olson. We taught them how to shoot and at one point or another, the better part of that group took me aside individually and asked how I was doing. When they were satisfied with my answer, they snatched my gun and started shooting.

What I'm trying to say — and forgive me if I use 100 words where 10 would have sufficed, I'm a writer and just as pompous as you can imagine — is that I appreciated everyone's good wishes. I appreciated their asking how I was doing and wishing me the best. But what I might have appreciated even more was their total awareness of the awkwardness of those very conversations. No one danced around the subject, no one tried to sugarcoat their own cancer stories even if the patient died.

No one tried to smoke me, in other words.

"Trey, heard you had cancer. How's that going? Good? Good. Feeling okay right now? Good, let's go get some pizza."

And for the entire weekend — shooting, signing books, talking with Jennifer Jordan about how her year was MUCH worse than mine, congratulating Jon and Ruth on the award for their fabulous magazine Crime Spree, meeting cool new people like the incredible Tribe, realizing just how much you loved old friends — that might well have been the highlight: not getting noticed for the First Aid kit from second grade.

It was a brilliant weekend and damn me if I didn't desperately need it.

Except now that I've written about swiping $$$ from Mama's purse, I'm sure she's gonna call me and demand that money back.

Comments

Mom, Oct 5, 2006

And we were poor as Job's turkey at the time! I won't dun you on *my* dime, kiddo. You'll have to assuage your guilt on *your* phone bill. Am really glad you were able to enjoy the convention so much, though. And I'll still send you a Christmas card this year.

Part 50: Wasting Away....
October 19, 2006 - 7:17 pm

Okay, not really wasting away, but WTF?

Went to the doc today. He was bored, which is good. He said all my counts look good; white blood cells are back up to a normal level of low, reds and platelets and everything else looks good. In other words, he was bored. (Actually, we spent the better part of the appointment talking about writing, which his daughter recently discovered and is very into.)

But — the caveat — I'm still losing weight!

For the last four days, I've been starving. Hungrier than I've been since last November when the good times started to roll right the fuck down hill. I've stuff myself with all kinds of food, scratched the itch, in other words. To the point where even LuAnn warned me to be careful. This from a woman who called me "old man skinny" more than once in the last few months.

I get there today and I'm at 166 according to their scale. Now, 166 ain't bad, ain't as bad as my home scale. Puts me down about 40/45 pounds. But I would have thought it was all coming back because I've been eating so much more recently.

When the nurse wasn't in the room, I snatched the chart, dashed down the hall, and made a copy.

12/8/05 (after a week of chemo and not eating), I was 200 pounds.

    12/15/05 — 195
    12/29/05 — 190
    1/26/06 — 189
    2/23/06 — 187
    4/20/06 — 180
    5/18/06 — 178
    6/9/06 — 173.5

7/13/06 — 171
7/20/06 — 170
9/7/06 — 169
10/19/06 — 166

A couple of interesting things in those numbers. First, according to their records, the weight didn't come off as fast as I thought I remembered. After that first 10 pounds down to 200, it went much slower than I realized. Secondly, I'm still exercising, growing muscle mass. My arms and legs are both way stronger than they used to be. So how is it I'm eating more, adding muscle, and still losing weight?

Officer Friendly — who stole me away for lunch today and never yelled at me about the amount I ate, but did look askance when that amount wasn't what he thought it should be — said I'm obviously not feeding the machine enough to counterbalance the exercise.

Here's the thing, though. I've gotten used to eating less and I like it. I like the weight I'm at, the way I feel. I don't want to get back into eating anything and everything in sight. So it'll be a delicate balancing situation. I need to eat a bit more for the exercising, but I don't want to gain a ton of weight, or the wrong kind of weight.

There isn't really a point to all of the above rambling, it's just where I am right now, forty-five days from the end.

Forty-five days! Makes me wanna giggle like a school girl. An entire year — actually slightly longer because of the surgery and whatnot — down to the last few breaths. Man, I can't even begin to explain how excited I am to be here.

Speaking of here, for any and all of you who might be in the area, December 4 is my chemo-free party. At the bookstore in Princeton. If you're around, pop in and have a Corona with me.

Comments

John P, Oct 19, 2006

Part 50! Jeeeeeez! But let the countdown to the last entry continue!

Y'know, there's a lot of research that suggests a low-calorie diet is extremely healthy. So if you're happy with the weight, let it settle into a comfortable spot and be one of the few thin Americans!

Too bad I'm near the wrong Princeton (NJ). Otherwise I'd be there.

Later…

Ellen D, Oct 19, 2006

You GO Trey!! Glad to hear you're doing so well.

Anonymous, Oct 21, 2006

That sounds like very good news. Congrats!

Part 51: The Final Countdown
November 2, 2006 – 8:58 pm

A few years ago, I was at a convention with Michael Arnzen. He's a hilarious poet and a damned scary writer. (Not that he personally is scary, though that's sometimes true, or that his writing is so bad it's scary, but that his books will scare you, I promise). He also is about the same age as me and we have quite a few of the same reference points in terms of movies and TV and music.

We're at this convention — Kansas City, I think it was — and the entire weekend, one of us sang "The Final Countdown" to the other. The song, if you remember, is Europe's only hit single and is one of those songs that once it gets into your head, it ain't going nowhere.

I hate that song.

But I like my own countdown.

Four weeks from today. Thirty-one days.

Fucking finally.

It's been tough, these last few weeks. The closer I get to being done, the harder it is to take the shot. I'll take them, in fact I might interrupt this writing session to go take one, it's getting to be about that time, and I'll take them to the bitter end, I'm just tired of them is all.

I realized a few days ago that things have changed. Where it was for so long lots of bad days with a few good moments buried beneath, then it was about 50/50 good days and bad, now it's much closer to a decent number of good days with a few bad moments buried beneath.

The hours after a shot are tough right now, I don't know why. But if I can get some sleep two or three hours after shooting up, I'm usually good to go the next day. I wonder, since the dosage is the same as it's been for weeks now, if that isn't at least partially psychological.

Seeing the end, can I take the process more easily? Could be.

Other than that, there is nothing going on. Counts are good, eating is good, weight is light but good, exercise is good. Just waiting out the last few weeks. Nothing else new or different to write about.

Actually, it's as boring as when I went to the doctor last week. Everything was so stable he was bored with me. I guess I'm starting to get bored with my treatment. Not annoyed like I have been, not angry or depressed, just bored.

That's okay, though, it's almost done.

Thirty one days. Thirty one days. Come on, baby, thirty one days.

Comments

Mike A, Nov 2, 2006

"Diddle-ee-doo. Diddle-ee-ee-doo. Diddle-ee-doo. Did-alee-ti-di-dee-doo, teeee-diddle-ee....diddleee...."

Gawd, I'm so sorry that's still ringing in your ears! It's unstoppable!

Hang in there, man. You're one of the strongest most patient people I know. And you make me the weirdo I am. I'm looking forward to seeing you again at another con soon (though let's hope it ain't Kansas City! Toronto in 2007?).

Mike Arnzen

ps – I don't think I ever told you: your book (2000 Miles to Open Road) puts John Woo to shame. Great fast-paced, noir, and entertaining novel!

Jared C, Nov 3, 2006

Now, see, I should've thought of John Woo.

And, excuse me, the ONLY hit Europe had? After repeated viewings of NickRocks at 6:30 after dinner, I can tell you that Europe produced the table-stomping "Rock the Night," the power ballad "Carrie" and the disappointing "Cherokee" (marching on the Trail of Tears…) off of the same album. Not to mention the follow-up "Superstitious" off the album of the same name. I'm FROM Texas!

I think I've just scared myself. I don't often get to use this limited amount of knowledge in my head, but now that I see it print, I don't know if I want to do it anymore.

Anyway, Trey, keep strong. Know that there are people thinking of you. And the Christmas season couldn't be a better time to celebrate the end.

In the meantime, I'll see if I can download some Europe Christmas music for ya.

Mikey Hyuck, Nov 11, 2006

I've been quietly reading your posts since we last talked, Trey, and watching you bounce from realization to realization like you're in slow-motion mosh. Besides it all being quite a fist-flailer, I expect you've shown many of the folks lining the pit what it's like on the inside when living with cancer. I know you taught me, and for that I'm grateful.

There's been a few times here, maybe within the last 90 days or so, where you mentioned the transition to boredom your doctor's taken. That, to me, is the most graphic of the mental pictures you drew. Probably because it's close, personally. I've seen it, yet I can't say I've ever heard any of the other folks I know with cancer or one of the other serious health challenges that'll give a person the same skewed divergent look at all the everyday, normal things in life. The things healthy folk take for granted. I've seen the bored doctor come and go, depending on the situation, and that by itself can be a stressor. Why is the {Oncologist for you, I s'pose, neurologist of me, ___ogist for someone else} concern and interest feigning or piquing sometimes, when I myself haven't shifted my own degree of giveadamn lately? Or the other way around…like when concern or frustration brings your own emotions to a fast boil, yet the doc remains mute and uninterested enough that you insist on searching his/her office for the rolling papers… For me, that one little aspect of the doctor's office visit was worse than even the wretchedly huge bills.

Between being a damn good writer and being a (ostensibly…hey, you know I dunno) damn good cop, I guess you were doomed to a life with sensitive senses. So seeing the boredom was to be expected. Reading it correctly, seeing it as substantiating the soundness of your health (which is how I read it, therefore how I'm able to unilaterally pronounce your reading "correct") is also, to me, a statement on your own state of mind. When you have the confidence to see yourself as relatively healthy, and getting healthier, well, I don't know how anyone could ask more from a patient. Other than to write less mystery and pick up a bit more horror. I could see how someone (such as myself) could ask you to do that. But then I've strayed off-subject, haven't I?

Take care of yourself, bro, and I'm looking forward to seeing you at the next convention we both can make. I'd like to try NeCon…I've never yet been there. Where's your next horror-related conventioneering gonna go down? Tell me…and perhaps we can get together and start a mosh.

Part 52: Of Old Men
Thursday, November 16th, 2006

So there's this old man, call him 157 years old. With perfectly coiffed Baptist/Televangelist/Texas Republican hair. It's all white and it never moved. He wore a blue track suit and I couldn't decide if he was a drug dealer or Pimp Daddy Old. Nice suit, though.

I was at the Princeton High School outdoor track, having decided to do my run outside rather than on a treadmill. Just something a little different, no big thing.

Yeah, piss on that. A huge different thing.

It sucked like a Hoover!

First of all, the track is much spongier than I'd realized so I felt like I was running in molasses. Had to work much harder to get any distance. Secondly, I had a headwind half the time, blowing cold-ass air into my face so I couldn't hardly breathe.

And, oh yeah, I had a chest cold! Hacking and wheezing and coughing up stuff that I wouldn't wish on my worst enemy. (I know, I know, don't run when you hurt, but I hadn't realized, until I started running, how severe the cold was).

So I'm running, managing to jog about half a lap, then walk half, then jog, etc. Quarter mile around the track so I'm not doing great. I'm not dead, but I'm not Carl Lewis, either.

Then this guy comes out of his house across the street, does a warm up or two, and starts jogging.

Son of a bitch never stopped! He was like a machine! Lap after lap after lap. Now, he wasn't jogging fast, but he wouldn't stop! Going slower than me but not having to walk half a lap.

Made me crazy. I just wanted this old dude to go home, stop making me look bad.

A lap or two around, he passed me, clapped his hand on my shoulder, and said, "Hang in there."

I could have killed him. It's one thing to watch him stomp me into the ground, another thing all together to get his pity while he does it.

What I'm going to do, see, is sneak into his house and muss up his perfect head'o'hair. Hah, that'll learn his ass!

***

This cold has left me in a strange position. I'm 16 days away from being finished with chemo (eight treatments, not that I'm counting) and I feel like I did back in January. I'm tired and weak, not hungry at all, cranky as hell, unmotivated to do anything. All the same things I had back in Jan when I started the home chemo project.

Or, The Home Chemo Project. Maybe I could sell that as some kind of reality show, make a few bucks on those of us throwing up and losing hair and all the other joys of chemo.

Extreme Home Makeover…Extreme Home Chemo.

Anyway, I find myself a little depressed by the current state. Yeah, yeah, I realize it's just a chest cold and it'll probably be gone in a few days, but I am what I am, I guess.

No great realization here or anything, just interesting that at the end, I am nearly as much of a mental wreck as I was at the beginning. The depression, minor though it is, feels exactly the same, like putting on a not-so favorite pair of ratty underwear because that's all there is left.

It's no problem, though. At least, not much of a problem. The depression is less than minor and in a few more days, a few more shots, all this mother-sucking, bullshitty crap will be over.

Booyah!

Part 53: Fucked it Up
Saturday, November 25th, 2006

So, I just spent something like an hour writing a new entry about the nostalgia of memory and how all I remember of last December — the worst month — was the brilliance of sleeping all the time; that I remember it fondly because I'm so tired now and have been for so long.

It was an incredible post, full of thoughtful words and images, of brilliant insight about the nature of memory and what not.

Then I screwed it. I'm two hours into a treatment and I'm as stupid as they come. I pushed some wrong button or whatever and poof!, the post disappeared.

And I'm too chemo stupid to rewrite it, at least right now. Maybe I'll try again later.

But the overriding thought is this: seven days from being finished. Only three more treatments.

Man, the computer screen is floating back and forth, reminds me of nothing so much as the Monkees movie. Head?

Was that the title?

Whatever.

Part 54: The Nostalgia of Memory
November 30, 2006 – 9:26 pm

Memory is a slippery thing.

Not only is it subject to the twists and turns of time, when we think we remember something one way and it turns out to be something else entirely (like thinking the movie "Ghost Story" was brilliant until I saw it again twenty years later), but also to interpretation.

Lately, I've been slipping into a nostalgia of last December, when all this started. All I can think about is how incredible the month was, how deeply fabulous, because the only responsibility I had was sleeping. Yeah, I had to get to the hospital, had to get the daily chemo, but really all I had to do was sleep.

God, for those days again.

I'm so tired right now that all I want to do is sleep. I want to crawl back to last December and sleep now as I did then.

Except that's not quite how the month went.

From *The Cancer Chronicles*, December 5, 2005

...the shakes are getting worse, but I have no muscle pain. I'm pretty sure that'll happen but maybe not until I'm driving down the highway at 80 or 90. hehehehe...okay, not particularly funny. For those of who you thought cancer would make me funnier, sorry....

...a bit of a thud across the top of my back, my thighs, and my calves a little....

From *The Cancer Chronicles*, December 19, 2005

...everything, except milk and orange sherbet, tastes like shit....

...Friday, Saturday, and a few minutes on Sunday saw me at the edge of passing out at odd, random moments. I get overheated very easily and then woozy and dizzy....

...the muddy brained? There seems to be nothing in particular that sets that off, it's just a general state right now. Sucks, though, because I can't remember anything and sometimes have a hard time putting together a sentence....

From *The Cancer Chronicles*, December 21, 2005

...most food tastes awful but even if it tasted good, I've got no appetite. And I'm sleeping the better part of 15 to 18 hours a day. When I'm awake, I'm weak, hardly able to walk up the stairs and even drag my ass to the bathroom to spit out a mouthful of white nastiness that, I suppose, is the Interferon....

...I'm having a hard time walking home from the hospital....

...I've had a fever most of the week. Standing in 17 degree weather wanting to do nothing so much as strip to the skin....

...the anger. I find I'm pissed all the time. Not like early on, when I joked about being mad at the whole concept of cancer. Now I'm furious. I don't want to deal with this bullshit....

So it wasn't just sleeping, it wasn't what I think I remember. It was harsh and ugly and tough. Why do I remember it differently? Because right now I'm exhausted and all I want to do is sleep. Some of that exhaustion is from the Interferon, some is from being so close to the end that I get frustrated and agitated.

But some of it is from work. In some sort of pathetic attempt to prove to everyone at work how tough I am, I took almost no vacation or sick time this entire year.

So that was a good plan, wasn't it? Yeah, yeah, I'm tough, I'm an Ironman...now can I have some time off?

Comments

Mom, Dec 1, 2006
    You have my permission to take off for a month!

Part 55: Finale
December 4, 2006 – 6:03 am

And so it's over.

And there was no revelation.

I had wanted to learn something, to have a great epiphany and discover some massive reserve of strength or vast store of single-mindedness; something that would make me believe I had become a better person, a more civilized or caring person, a more compassionate and loving person.

That was a large part of why I wrote *The Cancer Chronicles*, so that in the writing, I might polish a diamond out of a chunk of bullshit.

Squat.

When it was over, at 5:07 last night, it was just over.

Anticlimatically so, in fact. I gave the first shot, loaded up the second syringe, gave that shot, then tossed the entire works in the biohazard container. I stood up and announced to the deputies in the squad room that I was officially not dying of cancer anymore.

And that was that. No trumpets, no 3000 voice choir, no nude dancing girls.

Just...a shot...a shot...garbage.

Something that had begun with so much drama and pain, so much uncertainty and fear and anger, ended that easily. In fact, the end was almost boring in its banality.

I guess that's good. I guess flat and boring was better than the alternative, better than a repeat of the nightmare of November and December of 2005. Yeah, I could live without ever going through that bullshit again.

And yet, there was just a touch of drama at the very end. About a week ago, LuAnn made some off-hand comment to me.

I felt like crap — tired and cranky — and she said something like "If you hurt, just go to bed." But the tone was more along the lines of "Suck it the hell up already."

I knew that wasn't what she was saying, knew it in the core of my being, but I couldn't get it out of my head. I stewed all night, couldn't sleep at all. The next morning, angry and righteous and — more importantly — rock solid, I tried to tell her how the year had really gone.

But instead of solid, I fell apart...completely. Tried to tell her that it had been unfair of her to tell me to suck it up because she had no idea what I'd gone through. To prove my point, I heaped on her a pile of garbage so deep and wide and it left us both crying.

See, there were bad moments this past year, moments more terrible than I would have thought possible, much worse than what I told anyone. Eight or ten times, the light-headedness left me unconscious; one glorious time behind the wheel of my truck at a stop sign. I had felt it coming on and was racing home.

Didn't make it. Also didn't kill anyone, amazingly enough. There were vomiting sessions that went on for twenty/thirty/forty minutes and left me with nothing coming up but blood. One exercise session — when I was alone in the Princeton PD gym — I coughed so hard I got dizzy and passed out on the treadmill. Fell, banged my nose against the thing until there seemed to be blood everywhere, and skinned the hell outta my knee because the tread took a few seconds to stop.

There were nights where I was so scared I cried myself into a stupor.

There were times, especially after my biological father died of cancer in March, that I thought I was going to die. Nothing dramatic about it, just simple death. This is it, it'll be today. Or maybe tomorrow. But before the end of the week. I'll be dead and at least there won't be anymore hassles with the insurance company over the chemo.

And I never said a word.

THE CANCER CHRONICLES

LuAnn has had a hard year. Between worrying about me, trying to make sure there was money enough to buy the chemo, trying to run the bookstore with damned few days off because I simply couldn't work, she's had an absolutely shitty year. So I said nothing about the couple of times I went to the hospital or passed out on the toilet like a higher-rent Elvis.

I didn't want to worry her. I didn't want her carrying anymore baggage than what had already bent her back. As goofy as it sounds, I love her so much I didn't want to give her anything else. She didn't need anymore health bullshit from me. Cancer, the occasional bad back, and the heart attack, were more than enough.

At the same time, she hadn't said anything to me about how worried she actually was, how tired and scared. Because, she said in the middle of our cry-fest that left two feet of accumulated tears in the room, she didn't want to toss a few extra bodies on the grave yard of my worry.

Yes, we should have talked. Yes, we should have sat down and made sure each of us knew exactly what was going on with the other. But sometimes — most times, in fact — judgment is clouded by emotion.

But now it's over. I still have a bit of weakness and am still chemo-tired. And what in hell is my body going to think come Tuesday, when there is no shot? Shit, it'll be as shocked and probably scared as my colon was last December when all I could eat were salads and fruit.

Way back at the beginning of this, I wrote a Chronicle about the metaphor and how easy it was. I was in the middle of massive daily chemo and outside, the sun was hidden behind clouds while a foot of snow covered everything. I felt then that I was getting hammered in by everything, nature included.

Two days ago, 19 inches of snow pounded Princeton in something like five hours. Then the wind started to blow. The snow on my front yard was nearly two feet deep and it buried our two cars, one halfway up the driver's window.

This morning, mere hours after my last shot, I started digging. It was cold but the sun was out and blazing where it hadn't been a year ago. Unlike then, when I felt everything closing in around me, this morning, I was digging out.

Digging out. Literally. Metaphorically.

Completely and absolutely.

I think I'm gonna be okay.

Comments

Mom, Dec 4, 2006

You and LuAnn aren't the only ones who had a cry-fest this weekend. Yep, I think we let out our nerves, fears and "what-ifs" in all those tears. What a relief.

Debbie B, Dec 5, 2006

I received your ever personal mass email today and it reminded me that today is December and you're finished with chemo. I'm so glad you made it. I'm smiling just thinking about your ordeal being finished. I'm also trying to think of something funny and witty to say...nope, nothing is coming to mind – – just a quite prayer thanking our awesome God that he decided to let you live. Don't let him regret this decision.

Love always.

Bradley C, Dec 5, 2006

I truly deeply madly love you! Thank you for working so hard to stay with us. But then again, I know how fucking stubborn you are, so I know your ego wasn't about to let this shit take you down! Now go outside, face the sun, close your eyes, and just stand there and let the sun shine on your face for a while! (but know that a smile just might creep across your face when you do!)

With ALL my love and respect.

Tammy A, Dec 6, 2006

Sometimes in life there are road blocks, we just have to hit them head on. You and your family have done that. Now it is time to start living, go have a shot of your favorite beverage and scream out I BEAT YOU CANCER!!!!

I am so proud of you!

I love you, take care and stay healthy!

Dani D, Dec 9, 2006

Glad to hear you are cancer free. I suggest shots of Cabo for everyone. I had no doubt that you would beat this. If my memory serves me right you were always pretty stubborn.

Grandmother Smith, Dec 11, 2006

Dear Trey: I'm so happy it's over – I never doubted that with your grit and determination you would win this contest. Now you can get on with your life. Lots of love to you and LuAnn who has also fought her own battle.

Kelley C, Dec 26, 2006

Trey! Tonight I was playing around on the computer and "googling" like I usually do while my 3 year old watches Dora the Explorer, and I found you...or at least the website. I knew that you had been doing some writing and publishing, but had NO idea about the cancer! I just got finished reading your blogs and laughing my butt off at some of your comments. Where have I been? Why didn't I know about your writings and this battle against cancer?! I guess when we left Midland, we really did go our separate ways. I too am a cancer survivor....cervical cancer – clean now for the past 4 years! I'm so happy for you and your wife that things are turning around for you – at least health wise. I wish you the very best in 2007...I've got to put away the legos and get to the bookstore and checkout your books!

Trey, to Kelley C, Dec 31, 2006

Kelly, it's so great to hear from you. Wow, yet another cancer survivor. We should have our own survivor show. You know, running around a beach...okay, lounging around a beach, little drinks with umbrellas, cabana boys and girls waiting on us hand and foot.....

Seriously, it's great to hear from you and congrats on going four years clean, that's great. Please do drop me a line and let me know what else is up since we stumbled out of town different directions.

Tammy A to Kelley C, Jan 3, 2007

It's terrible to use someone else's misery to get in touch with the ones we have lost. Please email me and let me know what has been going on. I have sure missed our fun times together.

A Non Cancer Chronicle Update
December 31, 2006 – 7:38 pm

" - whatwashisnameanywayIthinkyoucan'tfindhim becausehe'sincustodyinGalesburgandwhataboutthat ThinToWinareyoudoingthatgoodluckyouknowifyouwanttolose weightyoucouldgoonthechemodietworkedformetothetuneof50p ounds – "

"Trey."

" – youknowI'vegotaweek'sworthofchemoinmy'fridgeit's yoursifyouwantitIthinkthecitydidagoodjobonthelightsthisyeargo t'emalluponthebuildingslookscoolhowwasChristmaseveryonege twhattheywantedprobablyallBattlestarGalacticaforyouI'llbet – "

"Trey. Shut up."

" – didItellyouI'mdonewithLauraBushnomoreFirstLady FantasiesabouthernomanshehadcanceranddiddidI'ttellanyoneuntil aftertheelectionsanditwasjusttooKarlRovianformedidtheythink peoplewouldn'tvoteforWifLaurahadcancersoI'mdonethinking aboutschtuppingtheFirstLadyontheWhiteHouselawnand — "

"Trey!"

"What?"

"Shut the hell up. I swear to God I'm going to shoot you in the head."

"What's the problem, big boy?"

"I'm not sure I can be your friend unless you go back on chemo."

Sadly, Officer Friendly isn't the only one who's said that. Most of my friends seem to prefer me on chemo. Basically, they're all saying, "Calm the frack down!"

Hehehehehehe.

I've got more energy than I know what to do with, is what's going on. The last bits of obvious chemo have finally slipped outta my system. I'm sleeping much more soundly (five or six solid hours a night rather than ten or twelve plagued hours), I'm eating well, I'm exercising everyday. I've got energy to burn baby.

And it's making my friends nutty. Which, of course, makes me laugh at them…as though I needed a reason.

I've gotten back to my writing, though I still have stamina problems because I still haven't refound the butt I lost during the weight loss. And most of the writing I've done on the new novel, about 25,000 words done while on chemo brain, doesn't suck as badly as I thought it might.

Work is going well. In fact, come February 18, I'll be headed off to the academy for twelve weeks in anticipation of being moved out of the jail and onto the road. So now, rather than being the guy who strip searches you after you get arrested, I'll be the guy who arrests you when you do terrible things to your dog with a fork.

(anyone get that reference?)

At the bookstore, I've managed to work quite a few days for LuAnn the last few weeks. Hell, she might've gotten more days off since Christmas than she got the entire year last year.

So things are going well right now. In fact, when they went this well back in the pre-cancer days, one of us would make a joke along the lines of, "Things are going too well, when is the brain tumor going to hit?"

Hahahahahaha…not quite so funny now.

I'm sitting here now, trying to think of what else to write about. There is nothing. Everything else is normal and my life is pretty boring. And yet, I've spent so much time cutting it open with a boning knife this past year, I feel like I should have something else interesting to say.

Nope.

So I guess that means I'm just like every other blogger out there, tapping madly away at the computer keyboard, somehow convinced that my life is interesting to anyone other than me. Quite the little conceit, don't you think?

Actually, I kind of wish that coffin salesman would call back. Now that I'm not quite so foggy brained, I might be able to keep up with him.

Comments

Scanner Darkly, Dec 31, 2006
>The fork reference: Steven Wright?

Aunt L, Jan 10, 2007
>Boy, it's a good thing you're not on cocaine – nobody would be able to stand you!

Cancer Chronicles Update
January 9, 2009 – 2:39 pm

So here we are, three years and a month since the madness (surgery, daily chemo, thrice weekly chemo, etc) began, and two years and a month since I celebrated the end of it all with friends, Dr Pepper, and massive amounts of Oreos.

I've been going to the doctor's office every three months since all this started. As I've gotten further away from it, the doctor has gotten more and more bored. To the point that for my last visit a few days ago, he didn't even show up. It was his assistant doctor.

That's pretty bored.

And by the by, my suggestions that, if he's so bored he should charge me half, have gone exactly no where.

But the point here, and the update, is that after three years, the doctor has put me on four month check ups rather than three. Small step, maybe, but an important one.

Statistically, with my kind of cancer, three years is a threshold. So getting past that is pretty good.

All the tests have been clean and positive and all the levels of various things are good and healthy and my weight has been stable and blah blah blah.

Yeah, I'll take the boring over the alternative.

But I still think I should get a discount of some sort.

Comments

Mom, Jan 11, 2009

Hurray for passing the 3-year hurdle! No matter what you tell yourself, you still think about it.

Congrats!

Oh, yeah, you certainly *should* get a discount. Dumb system.

Afterword

It's December 24, 2009 as I write this. The air is full of Christmas. There is snow on the ground, as there was when I started this odyssey way back when. It's raining and it's cold and I'm not sure when the last time I saw the sun was. I've got Dr. John playing – his brilliant *Anutha Zone* album. Most notably, I'm alive, I'm cancer-free, I'm fairly good looking, in a roguish sort of way, and I've got a killer sense of humor.

Okay, obviously, two of those four things aren't true. I'll let you decide which.

Since *The Cancer Chronicles* ended, I've had a number of people discover them. Sometimes it's newly found friends, sometimes it's old friends I've not spoken to in years. But every once in a while, I get emails from people trolling the internet for items on cancer.

Because they have the shit.

They've had the same meeting with a doctor or two or three that I had and they're going through all the same shit I did. Maybe they're strong and ready to get down to battle, or maybe they're still crying and trying to adjust to their new title in life, 'Cancer Patient,' or maybe they're curious because a loved one is dealing with it.

Sometimes those people email me. Not very often and it's never earth-shattering when they do. They don't tell me I've saved their life or changed their life or anything even remotely like that.

Usually, they laugh at me.

They laugh because I fell in the street. They laugh because the coffin salesman tried to sell me something I definitely didn't need. They laugh at the Gummi Bears or orange sherbet or whatever. It's a nervous sort of laughter but it is laughter, even in emails, and that's good enough for me.

Telling these stories helped me get through a life's worth of bullshit. And telling them as I lived them gave them an immediacy that I don't often match in my writing. I love these stories, as hard and brutal and funny and goofy as they are, and hopefully you did, too. And if they make you laugh and help you get through your own life's worth of bull snot, then so much the better.

When I was putting this book together, I never thought of skipping the comments. So many of them are full to bursting with their own insight and heartache, I had to include them. They were an integral part of what I went through and so frequently renewed my faith in my particular world that they couldn't be edited out.

But I did have a problem with formatting them. Some comments were from friends who signed with just their first names. Some were from people I vaguely knew who signed with their full names. Some included only their email addresses. Still others were from people I didn't know at all. 'Kylie' is a good example. I have no idea who she was and I've not heard from her since.

What I chose to do was list people by their first names and first letter of last name, sort of an old-fashioned literary device that I've always found interesting. For those with no last name, their first name is all you see. For those who never left a name, I listed them as 'anonymous,' which is how they came up on my blog. For those who signed with email addresses, that's what you get. I tried to keep all that as plain and clear as I could. But I had to have some kind of name for them. I wanted, if at all possible, for you to come to know them as personally as I had.

So it's been four years since diagnosis, almost four years since the month of hellish daily treatments ended, and three years since I finished it all and celebrated with booze and cookies. I'm still going to the oncologist and probably will be for life, but he's still bored and I'm still glad of it.

And though I enjoyed – if I can use that word – writing these chronicles, I'd rather not have any updates. Dr. John has a line in one of the *Anutha Zone* songs that I've always used as sort of touch point for the characters in my fiction.

"I just wanna dream better, no more nightmares."

Right now, I'm dreaming pretty good.

Bonus Track:

Mid-February, 2001
(Originally published in *Cemetery Dance*)

February 18, 2001.
About 9:00 am.
I'm in a shop, overseeing the building of a set I designed for a musical. Lots of noise, lots of dust, lots of paint. It's a gray day, overcast with clouds looking like nothing so much as late term pregnant women. I hope they give birth, I love the rain.

This is the first of three shows I'll be working on during this one day. Three different shows, three different theaters, sixteen hours with no scheduled break.

I did this to myself.

***

From: <DickLaymon>
To: <TreyRBarker>
Sent: Saturday, February 10, 2001, 11:24 AM
Subject: Re: First Novel Blurb
Hi, Trey --
Very good idea to do up your first chapter as a chapbook and send it around to conventions for the goodie bag. I'd be glad to read your mystery and give it a blurb.

Best,
Dick

***

February 18, 2001
About 11:00 am.

I've left the shop and am sitting in front of Temple Events Center. My little Ford Ranger is crammed with audio and light gear. Amps, mixers, PA speakers, a CD player, cables, lights galore, dimmer packs, more cables, colored gels, computerized light board, tools. Lunch.

My truck sits way back on its rear axle. It looks like a fairly straight laced 34 year old white boy trying desperately to be hip with a low-slung truck.

It isn't raining yet but will any minute. The rain is so thick I can smell it. I grew up in west Texas where it rained once a year whether it needed to or not. I can't wait, I love the rain.

I begin unloading the mountain of gear. It's for a dance show that is raising funds for the earthquake victims in India. They've been hit twice in only weeks and it's hard for me to imagine going through something so life changing. I can't imagine anything other than the safe, comfortable life I lead. A little chaotic sometimes but a good life, filled with the knowledge that everything will always be fine.

***

A paraphrase of a phone conversation on February 12 or 13, 2001:

Trey: "...damned thing ain't working for shit."

Dick: "You know, sometimes when I get stuck, I go to the end. Write that last scene and then see what you need directly before it and write that. Then go right before that scene and write that."

Trey: "Oh, that's freakish, I never thought of that."

Dick: "If that doesn't work for you, send me the manuscript and I'll give it a read. Maybe I can figure out what's wrong with it."

Trey: "I don't know, I've fucked it up pretty good."

Dick: "I'm sure it's fine, it's just hard to see sometimes when you're that close to a project."

***

February 18, 2001
About 11:15 am.

At first, I thought it was pollution. Denver had had three days' worth of a temperature inversion. Our brown cloud would have made even LA envious. Then I thought maybe it was because I was unloading all that audio and light equipment. Lots of unloading, lots of physical exertion. Had to be one of those two things, didn't it? This shortness of breath couldn't be anything serious. Hell, I'm only 34, what else could it be?

It still wasn't raining and I realized, as the first pains thudded through the middle of my chest, that the lack of rain was bumming me out. I wanted to see some rain.

I called 911 real quick. In fact, my Texas homeboys will probably take away my Texas Native Membership Card when they find out I didn't tough out the pain.

The ambulance was there within five minutes. Then I was on the ground, staring at the sky -- still no rain -- and trying to tell the paramedics what was wrong with me. I think I may have mentioned something about having two heads and three arms. I don't remember much of that conversation.

I just remember the pain.

***

From: <Tom Piccirilli>
To: <TreyRBarker>
Sent: Wednesday, February 14, 2001, 2:54 pm
Subject: Fwd: Laymon
Received this from Ed Gorman a few minutes ago.
<< Dick Laymon died two hours ago of a heart attack. >>

***

I didn't see Dick when I had my heart attack, but he was there.

There was no apparition of Dick in the corner or floating over my bed or standing behind the nurses. But he was in my head. I was hypersensitive to heart attacks because of Dick. I called 911 more quickly than I probably would have because of Dick. I was in the hospital, IVs and EKGs, making bad jokes at the nurse's expense (memo: don't make jokes about a woman holding lots of needles while she's trying to save your life, it's bad form) because of Dick.

My quick recovery is not a silver lining, there is no silver lining in death.

But Dick's death did make me think. It did make me call 911 quickly.

Dick's death did help me, though it shreds my insides to say that. Seems like a high price to pay for me to have suffered a mild heart attack instead of a massive heart attack.

***

Dick and I became -- I like to think, anyway -- quite good friends over the last year. Mutual friends -- Tom Piccirilli, Alan Beatts - brought Dick and I together, though I'd been a fan of his work for years. He and I talked frequently about writing and publishing and similar topics that were oh so heavy and deeply thought out and full of philosophy. But after that, like a cheap beer after an expensive meal, we talked about the kind of stupid, inane bullshit that so often seems to fill phone conversations.

But it is those very stupid things that made me realize Dick was more than just a writer spending lots of his own time helping younger writers. It was those things that made me realize Dick was simply a cool guy and would have been cool whether spending his life writing or clerking in a low-rent convenience store in south-central LA.

Obviously, I will miss him.

Obviously, the world of literature will miss him.

There is no silver lining, but he helped me. And maybe my heart attack can help someone else. In a strange way, a perverse and dark way that Dick might have chuckled over, it's what Dick had been doing for years.

By the way, it still hasn't rained.

www.ingramcontent.com/pod-product-compliance
Lightning Source LLC
Chambersburg PA
CBHW020912290526
45784CB00002BA/515